BEING HUMAN

EDITED BY
ALASTAIR MORGAN

BEING HUMAN

REFLECTIONS ON MENTAL DISTRESS IN SOCIETY

EDITED BY
ALASTAIR MORGAN

PCCS BOOKS
Monmouth

First published in 2008
Reprinted 2009, 2015

PCCS Books Ltd
Wyastone Business Park
Wyastone Leys
Monmouth
NP25 3SR
UK
Tel +44 (0)1600 891 509
www.pccs-books.co.uk

This collection: © Alastair Morgan, 2008

Introduction © Alastair Morgan, 2008; Chapter 1 © John Cromby, 2008;
Chapter 2 © Philip Thomas, 2008; Chapter 3 © Ian Parker, 2008;
Chapter 4 © Alastair Morgan, 2008; Chapter 5 © Miles Clapham, 2008;
Chapter 6 © Helen Spandler, 2008; Chapter 7 © Susannah Wilson, 2008;
Chapter 8 © Jocelyn Catty, 2008; Chapter 9 © Christopher D. Ward, 2008;
Chapter 10 © Patrick Callaghan, 2008; Chapter 11 © David R. Wilson, 2008;
Chapter 12 © Robert Diamond, 2008; Chapter 13 © David Smail, 2008.

All rights reserved.
No part of this publication may be reproduced, stored in a retrieval system, transmitted or utilised in any form by any means, electronic, mechanical, photocopying or recording or otherwise without permission in writing from the publishers.
The authors have asserted their rights to be identified as the authors of this work in accordance with the Copyright, Designs and Patents Act 1988.

Being Human: Reflections on mental distress in society

A CIP catalogue record for this book is available from the British Library

ISBN 978 1 906254 06 3

Cover design by Old Dog Graphics
Printed by Lightning Source, Milton Keynes, UK

CONTENTS

Introduction   1
Alastair Morgan

PART ONE: UNDERSTANDING AND REPRESENTING MENTAL DISTRESS

1. Feelings, Beliefs and Being Human   12
   John Cromby

2. Towards a Critical Perspective on 'Narrative Loss' in Schizophrenia   24
   Philip Thomas

3. Constructions, Reconstructions and Deconstructions of Mental Health   40
   Ian Parker

4. The Authority of Lived Experience   54
   Alastair Morgan

5. Philosophy and Psyche: What can philosophy tell psychiatry, psychology and psychotherapy?   71
   Miles Clapham

PART TWO: SYMPTOMS IN SOCIETY

6. The Radical Psychiatrist as Trickster   84
   Helen Spandler

7. Writing from the Asylum: A re-assessment of the voices of female patients in the history of psychiatry in France   99
   Susannah Wilson

8. Mirrors of Shame: The act of shaming and the spectacle of female sexual shame 110
    Jocelyn Catty

9. Symptoms in Society: The cultural significance of fatigue in Victorian Britain 125
    Christopher D. Ward

10. Artaud's Madness: The absence of work? 138
    Patrick Callaghan

PART THREE: CRITICAL REFLECTIONS ON PRACTICE

11. A Phenomenological Encounter: Prelude to a mental health assessment in a magistrate's cells 151
    Dave R. Wilson

12. Opening up Space for Dissension: A questioning psychology 174
    Bob Diamond

13. Clinical Psychology and Truth 190
    David Smail

Contributors 197

Index 201

ACKNOWLEDGEMENTS

I would like to thank all the contributors for their time and effort in helping to produce the volume, and Pete Sanders at PCCS Books for his support and patience with the project. Particular thanks must go to Tim Calton, who was the key figure in organising the seminar series and bringing together the participants who have contributed to this volume. Thanks should go to Nottinghamshire NHS Trust and the School of Nursing Research Group at the University of Nottingham for their assistance in the funding of the seminar series from which this book arose.

Above all, I would like to thank Marion for her continued love, encouragement and support.

INTRODUCTION

ALASTAIR MORGAN

The contents of this book originated in a series of seminars presented between 2005 and 2007 at the University of Nottingham under the auspices of the HUMAN research project, which was funded by a Managed Innovation Network grant from Nottinghamshire NHS Trust.

The HUMAN research group consisted of a broad range of academics, practitioners in the mental health field, service users and carers, all with an interest in issues at the interface between mental health, mental distress and the humanities, broadly conceived. Our aims were fundamentally and determinedly eclectic. We hoped to encourage reflection from fields in the humanities (philosophy, history, psychology, literature) in order to stimulate debate about the nature of mental distress in society. Although our shared ethos was one of a broad critique of a narrowly biological conception of psychiatry, we didn't set out with any political programme or manifesto, nor were we attempting to tie ourselves to the constraints of clinical or empirical relevance. Indeed, we hoped that the encouragement of a broad agenda, and a mixed audience, would facilitate an experience of debate and education that would enable interesting and felicitous connections to arise.

Throughout the two years of the seminar series, we managed to attract a diversity of speakers and audiences from across the academic disciplines, from a variety of mental health professions, and users of mental health services and their carers, although, of course, these groupings are not discrete and will always cross over. This book represents a strong cross-section of the themes and participants of those seminars. However, what cannot be easily represented within the covers of a book is the intellectual space that was created within the seminar series, even for a short period of time. In a professional and academic field driven by targets, evidence and outputs, the ability of people to just take a breath and reflect in an atmosphere of genuine enquiry and dialogue came as a relief to many participants, including those based within academic settings which one would think would be set up primarily for this purpose. It is this space to think about what mental distress is, its place in society, and the relation that psychiatry has to mental distress that was particularly invigorating in such an environment and became the inspiration for this book.

PSYCHIATRY DOESN'T THINK

In his foreword to the 1997 translation of Karl Jaspers' seminal conceptual work in psychopathology, *General Psychopathology*, originally written in 1913, Paul McHugh relates an encounter between Jaspers and one of his psychiatric colleagues in a meeting. Jaspers is reported to have said, 'To make real progress psychiatrists must learn to think', and his colleague is reported to have replied 'Jaspers ought to be spanked' (McHugh, 1997: vii).

If we take psychiatry to be the name for a broad tradition of mental health care and practice (inclusive of psychology, nursing, social work etc.), we could still wonder what it means for psychiatry, as this broad discipline, to reflect upon its conceptual foundations. Of course, in some sense, an unthinking postmodern pragmatism will argue that the kind of grand conceptual scheme exemplified by books such as *General Psychopathology* is a product of the overweaning arrogance of enlightenment thought that should be dispensed with in favour of local knowledges and practices. However, the reluctance to reflect upon the conceptual bases and meanings of the discipline of psychiatry leave it open to the kind of meaningless models of governmental best practice that mix an unholy mess of increasing compulsion, medication, certain forms of therapy and ideologies of social inclusion that themselves remain unthought in relation to each other. Thus, we are all instructed to adopt principles of recovery and social inclusion as the core practices in mental health care, whilst at the same time a new Mental Health Act restricts the amount of freedom and choice available to those most in need within the mental health system.

One of the ways of trying to think what psychiatry is and should be is to reflect upon its position as a crucible between the humanities and, what used to be termed, the natural sciences. Jaspers' great achievement, almost a century ago, was the adoption of such a position for psychiatry as a virtuous starting point for the discipline. For Jaspers, if psychiatry was to develop as a tradition, it needed to stake its claim as a discipline that was concerned both with the methodologies of the natural sciences (explanation according to cause and effect), and understanding as the method appropriate to the human sciences (the empathic grasping of the meaningful connections of human life as a whole). Of course, this attempt to stake a position on the fence, to speak in a crass manner, caused as many problems as it solved. This is why I refer to this position for psychiatry as a kind of crucible, a place of strife rather than a happy home. This place of strife continued throughout the twentieth century, with the contestations over the nature of mental distress, its treatment and the proper place for psychiatry as a discipline. Mainstream psychiatry took its place within a medical paradigm, but remained a permanent shameful cousin, because of its lack of any objective identifiable organic causation for mental illness, and its constant reshaping and restructuring of its own central categories and claims. On top of this, was the inevitable entanglement of psychiatry with the worst practices of twentieth century totalitarianism, which meant that by the late 1960s and 1970s, psychiatry as a discipline was under sustained pressure and attack, alongside many of the other central disciplines and institutions of Western capitalist societies.

In a sense, psychiatry survived such a radical contestation and prospered as a medical discipline with the conservative backlash against radical movements in the 1980s and

1990s, but as we move into the new century, psychiatry as a tradition, a tradition that attempted to think its central conceptual foundations, seems to be withering on the vine. It may well be that the twenty-first century will see psychiatry disappear as a discipline, as it fragments into a number of sub-specialities, and as it eats its own diagnostic categories, only for them to be functionalised as specific behavioural disorders. For example, the concept of schizophrenia, a concept under sustained attack and interrogation since its inception, may well eventually be abolished, only to be replaced by a series of discrete functional descriptions of various psychotic behaviours (i.e. delusional, anxiety, or drug-induced psychosis). In the movement from the grand modernist concept of schizophrenia to the localised knowledges of functional disorders, we come no closer to the meaningful interpretation of the lifeworld of the person existing in a psychotic state.

In a paper entitled, 'Madness, the Absence of Work', Michel Foucault speculates, in a rather ambivalent way, about the possibility of the disappearance of madness as a category from the social scene. He writes that:

> Perhaps some day we will no longer really know what madness was. Its face will have closed upon itself, no longer allowing us to decipher the traces it may have left behind. (Foucault, 1995: 290)

For Foucault, this appears to be a loss, in the sense that madness is an integral category for attempting to decipher certain ways of being and understanding in society, but, at the same time one will be rid of all the romantic misattributions that the term attracts. We could supplement Foucault's argument with the disappearance of that great twentieth century other of madness, psychiatry, in all its diversity and its inglorious history. Perhaps both madness and psychiatry will disappear together. The attempt to understand that which is beyond understanding, that should be, and at times is, at the centre of the tradition of psychiatry, will disappear. What will replace it is already apparent in outline. There will be a series of practices of manipulating and improving the human psyche, within an increasing framework of mental health and well-being that focuses on the continuum of mental experiences and on a hybrid of techniques, both pharmacological and therapeutic, that can optimise human potentialities defined in terms of functioning. The whole project of understanding the mad is completely incidental to such a new formulation, as are the central conceptual underpinnings of any self-reflective tradition of psychiatry. Indeed, the concept of a psychopathology becomes redundant in the sense that the pathological has no meaning any more when the purpose of mental health care is to focus on the population as a whole, rather than to simply isolate certain abnormal members of society. Nevertheless, practices of compulsion and coercion remain, but their centrality as the ethical problem in mental health care becomes sidelined and occluded by an ideology of mental well-being that wants to produce happiness as a functional requirement of productive citizenship in a modern society.

With the disappearance of psychiatry, positive outcomes would be numerous. One would hope to see a lessening of stigma around experiencing mental health problems, alongside an acceptance of mental health problems, as caused by biological predispositions, however conceptualised, rather than weakness of character. However, given the current configurations of mental health services and practice it seems unlikely that the central tensions that initially animated psychiatry would have any place in these new configurations. I think a return to these tensions could enlighten us when trying to think of a place for a different kind of psychiatry for the twenty-first century, a psychiatry that would be nourished through reflection on the overlap between mental health care and the humanities.

JASPERS' FIVE HORIZONS FOR AN UNDERSTANDING OF PSYCHIATRY

In the introduction to *General Psychopathology*, Jaspers lists what he terms fundamental horizons, within which 'our psychic realities present themselves' (Jaspers, 1997: 6). These are the five central concepts of psychiatry; the fundamental and basic categories of psychiatry. However, as the word 'horizon' suggests, they are not clearly delineated foundational concepts, but rather central problems or areas of tension that situate and orientate the practice of psychiatry as a discipline at the crossroads between the human and the natural sciences. For Jaspers, these central questions for psychiatry are central questions of what it means to be human, and it is only through an enquiry into the meaning of being human that we can understand mental distress.

First, Jaspers states that the object of study in psychopathology is the human, and that we need to be aware of the specific and interesting differences between human animals and non-human animals when discussing psychopathology. Whereas medicine treats physical illness as a model that applies to animality as a whole, when we are dealing with mental distress we are interested in a phenomenon particular and peculiar to human animals. Even in her physical embodiment, the human animal has important differences from non-human animals through the expressive uses of her body. Therefore, first and foremost, mental distress should be related to the particular potentialities of human freedom. This does not mean that we are not bound to the necessities of our physical incarnations, but that we have also to carve out a meaning for our life, and that fundamentally being human, therefore, is a dual incarnation of both vulnerability and incompleteness, and these are the key factors to explore when looking at mental distress. Jaspers writes:

> [T]he concept of human psychic illness introduces a completely new dimension. Here the incompleteness and vulnerability of human beings and their freedom and infinite possibilities are themselves a cause of illness. (Jaspers, 1997: 8)

Furthermore, humans form societies and cultures and have their own self-understandings that should be taken into account whenever we consider mental distress. Mental distress is a product of being human, in the sense of human incompleteness and vulnerability, and in the sense that it takes place within a specific historical, social and cultural milieu.

The second basic concept or horizon for psychiatry is the problem of, what Jaspers terms, the 'objective manifestation of psychic life' (Jaspers, 1997: 9). By this, he means that we cannot understand the psychic life of a person as though it were an object or a fact, and in its manifestation it is always unclear and occluded. We only understand another person through their speech, and physical gestures and expressiveness. When this is even more alien, as in the case of severe mental distress, then we have further difficulties of interpretation, of trying to grasp and understand the phenomena of psychic life. When we are trying to do this, what we are doing is attempting to grasp, not a fact or a thing, but a process that is continually unfolding, and that is never finally achieved. With this horizon for psychiatry, Jaspers is instigating the central difficulties of what it means to understand the life of another person, and particularly, how we can understand the life of someone who is severely mentally distressed and thus cannot easily communicate their psychic life.

Third, what we are concerned with, when confronted with human distress, is a conscious being, a being that is aware of its self, aware of its experience, and its surroundings. However, we should try and distinguish between conscious and unconscious experience, or what Jaspers sometimes terms 'extra-conscious' experience, which will include for him, both unconscious drives and memories, and biological and physical mechanisms.

Fourth, there is the relation between what Jaspers terms the inner and the outer. What he means here is the way in which psychic life becomes recognised and taken up within a social and environmental world. To adapt a phrase from Heidegger, we could call this the mode of 'being-in-the-world'. This is in the sense of how we are always as humans engaged in the world, and also how our environment and the situations we find ourselves within can foster our own growth and feeling of selfhood within the world. An understanding of human mental distress can only occur through an understanding of how this process of recognition and mutual incorporation of environment and psyche occurs within an individual.

Finally, Jaspers argues that psychiatry should be concerned with what he terms 'the differentiation of psychic life'. This is perhaps the most obscure of Jaspers' central concepts, and one would have to admit that the descriptions he gives of it are not particularly helpful, and even fundamentally flawed (for example, the references to the 'furthest evolved' illuminating the primitive, see Jaspers, 1997: 13). However, I think this is best explained as an argument for an understanding of the cultural forms of objectification of psychic life. We can only truly understand what it means to be human, and correlatively, what it means to experience mental distress, if we understand the multiple ways of living different forms of life. Jaspers clearly means differentiation to refer to what could be loosely termed a level of intellectual development, as well as this argument about cultural milieu, although I think that this is not particularly helpful. However, a generous interpretation of what he says here would state that human psychic life can only be understood through an understanding of its historical and cultural incarnation.

To summarise these five central concepts for psychiatry, as concepts that psychiatry must think in all its endeavours:

1. The particularity of human existence, in its incompleteness and vulnerability.
2. The problem of how we can gain access to individual's thoughts, emotions and feelings, particularly as they are not objects, but processes.
3. What we are concerned with are conscious beings with their own self-understandings. But any consciousness also has unconscious and extra-conscious elements. What, then, is the relationship between these different factors?
4. Any understanding of human mental distress has to understand it as unfolding within a relationship to a specific situation and environment.
5. That situation and environment does not only have an individual relevance, but also a societal and cultural milieu, which allows for the differentiation of human forms of life, and needs to be taken into account as fundamental in any understanding of mental distress.

'JASPERS IS IN THE BIN'

I would argue that these five questions or horizons as central organising principles for psychiatry are still as relevant today as they were for Jaspers.[1] We may well reformulate the language, and want to answer them in significantly different ways, but as an orientation for the enterprise of psychiatry, they still seem a comprehensive starting point for any attempt, not only to understand, but to explain mental distress. Therefore, to try and explain mental distress through a straightforward procedure of brain imaging, and pointing to certain images of the lighting of different portions of the brain, is not going to, in itself, negotiate any of the questions that Jaspers raises. What we need is to try and understand such neuroscience in relation to the central questions of what it means to be a conscious human living in the world. Furthermore, to abstract certain functional cognitive capacities and then investigate them as discrete entities, or facts of psychic life, will never give us an understanding of what it means to be in the terms of a continual, incomplete and vulnerable process of developing as a human being.

However, it seems that many dominant strands of psychiatric practice and research do not want to think through these central questions. We are left with a psychiatric research paradigm that emphasises the accumulation of evidence based on facts, and fetishes technology to the extent of reputable studies having to be accompanied by their

---

[1]. I am aware that this argument for a 'return to Jaspers' puts me in conflict with some of the other contributors to this volume. For example, Philip Thomas and Patrick Bracken have cogently argued that Jaspers' outlook is tied to a Cartesian worldview and therefore constrained by a methodological individualism. I agree with some of their central claims, but still think that Jaspers' framing of the central questions and problems for psychiatry makes sense and has relevance. See Bracken & Thomas, 2005: 117–22.

requisite trundling of patient groups through the favourite brain imaging technique.

On the other hand, we have what I term a postmodern pragmatism, which stresses that there are no truths out there, and that there is no *telos* of progress just a pragmatic negotiation of checks and balances, and that we should be sceptical of any grand themes or metanarratives.

All of this results in the dissolution of the central concepts of psychiatry into the burgeoning ideology of mental well-being. An anecdote may bring this home. For over a year, I had borrowed a very old copy of Jaspers' *General Psychopathology* from a major medical library. Eventually, I decided to return it (needless to say, it hadn't been requested by anyone else). Six months later, I returned to the library to try and borrow it again, to find that it had disappeared from the catalogue. On asking the library staff, I found that it had been remaindered. Jaspers was in the bin.

BEING HUMAN

The contents of this volume return to these five central questions, and attempt to shed a new and different light on the intersections between the humanities and mental health.

In part one, 'Understanding and Representing Mental Distress', contributors reflect upon the central problems of how to understand mental distress as a particular way of being human, and the problem of trying to understand and give a voice to mental distress.

In 'Feelings, Beliefs and Being Human', John Cromby gives an account of embodiment and feelings as central to any interrogation of what it means to be human. Such an interrogation takes into account an argument for feelings as an already socialised yet pre-reflective and ineffable basis for all our beliefs. Cromby importantly integrates an idea for an embodied basis for human being, alongside that basis being socially produced, by arguing that this embodied basis is already socially mediated by the time we try to reflect upon it and grasp it. Through reflections on a published history of mental distress, he articulates an account of how feelings can lie at the basis of delusional beliefs.

Philip Thomas reflects on what it means to understand severe mental distress, and what it means for someone to give an account of that distress. He questions the predominance of narrative representation within much of the literature in philosophy and psychiatry and argues for an attention to different forms of expression and interpretation. Crucially, he refers to the meaning that can lie in the absence of words or the gaps in attempts to express inner states.

In his chapter entitled 'Constructions, Reconstructions and Deconstructions of Mental Health', Ian Parker tackles the question of representation at a conceptual rather than an individual level. Through interrogating the concept of mental health in its cultural specificity, he argues for a deconstruction of the concept that can open us to the forces at play in its deployment. He argues, significantly, for a hermeneutic practice of attempting to excavate what is hidden and suppressed in any account of mental health, and by analysing cultural and media discourses around mental health he demonstrates how the concept of mental health is deployed as a tracing of the boundaries between normality and pathology.

In my chapter, 'The Authority of Lived Experience', I question the concept of lived experience as it is used in qualitative accounts of mental distress. I explore the conceptual history of the concept of lived experience and draw out three strands to the concept, which need to be interrogated in any account of a person's lived experience.

In 'Philosophy and the Psyche', Miles Clapham explores the limits of understanding and communication within therapeutic encounters, through a reflection on Wittgenstein's philosophy.

This opening section of the book revolves around how to understand mental distress in its specificity as cultural phenomenon and in its continuity with human life as a whole, without suppressing its difference. Importantly, all of the contributions share a concern with a hermeneutic practice that is alert to meaning that remains concealed or unspoken, or hard to express in one form or another.

In the second part of the book, entitled 'Symptoms in Society', contributors interrogate what it means to experience mental distress or critically interrogate mental distress as a cultural and historical form of life. These contributions are concerned with an analysis of mental distress that only arises through its construction and appearance within a specific historical and cultural milieu. Rather than treating symptoms of mental distress as an ahistorical fact, these symptoms are inserted back into their societal context.

Helen Spandler offers an account of critiques of psychiatry as themselves tied to powerful tensions and contradictions stemming from the societal forms in which they arise. Through an analysis of 'trickster' figures in general, and of Julian Goodburn's critical practice at the Paddington Day Hospital in the 1970s in particular, she locates a paradoxical position for those figures who incarnated both a critique of psychiatry and an authoritative figure in their own right. Furthermore, she reflects upon how narratives of these figures can suppress their importance and critical edge by means of erasing their radical attempts from any genuine history of psychiatry. The 'trickster' figure should be interrogated as an emblem of contradictions and tensions that lie at the very heart of any attempt to change psychiatric practice in a certain place and time.

Susannah Wilson is also concerned with reconstructing hidden narratives in her chapter, which interprets and presents accounts from women incarcerated in asylums in nineteenth century France. She provides a powerful interpretation of these accounts of delusional beliefs as symbolic narratives of resistance to real life oppression and suppression of women's lives in a particular society. Her methodology is to engage with the delusional content itself as particularly meaningful and understandable in the context of the life history of the person as a whole.

Jocelyn Catty interrogates the oscillation between concealment and exposure exemplified in shame and acts of shaming through an analysis of Elizabethan poetry. Through a careful deployment of her literary sources, she outlines the interrelationship between representation and shame, and draws important parallels with the therapeutic encounter, by questioning how we can represent another person's mental distress without entering into an act of shaming.

The central chapter of this section, from which the whole section takes its name, is Chris Ward's 'Symptoms in Society', in which he offers a fascinating and powerful comparison between one outmoded psychiatric diagnosis and one very current diagnosis, namely those of neurasthenia and chronic fatigue syndrome. He locates neurasthenia as a set of symptoms that arose within a particular constellation of ideas and forces at the end of the nineteenth century. By interrogating cultural and philosophical accounts of energy and fatigue, he gives a powerful account of neurasthenia as a symptom that could only arise given its cultural and societal milieu, and then raises similar considerations regarding chronic fatigue syndrome. Importantly, this is not an exercise in philosophical idealism, but a way of arguing for both a biological basis and a societal and cultural basis for symptoms. Ward wants to emphasise that the history of symptoms in psychiatry is always both an aspect of the history of ideas as well as the history of diseases, and that any symptom can only be fully understood given its societal and cultural background.

This section is concluded by Patrick Callaghan's reflections upon the figure of Antonin Artaud, in the light of the paper I have already cited by Foucault, namely 'Madness and the Absence of Work'. Callaghan offers an account of differing views of what madness and health mean, and articulates a space in which madness is both produced by the absence of work, but also in a sense defined by such an absence. Artaud becomes the emblematic figure of such a space, and his life work oscillates between madness as an absence of work and as a catalyst for work.

In the final section of the book, three contributions offer critical reflection on practice in mental health. How can we both be critical and still offer a practice that can help people? Dave R. Wilson interrogates the problem of what it means to be non-judgemental through a radical account of the attempt to adopt a non-judgemental attitude prior to even talking with someone. He gives a detailed phenomenological account of the performance of a non-judgemental stance in a highly controlled setting, namely a magistrate's cells. Wilson articulates the tensions involved in the attempt to achieve a posture of tranquil receptivity with verve and power.

Bob Diamond directly confronts the issue of what it means to be critical and helpful, through the adoption of a framework that emphasises social factors in the production of mental distress, and argues for a way of doing psychology that attempts to move away from a methodological individualism towards taking account of the material and social factors that determine people's lives.

Finally, David Smail offers a critical perspective on the current status of discourse in the mental health sphere, and an acute analysis of the power and vested interests at play within the mental health professions. He argues against the pernicious dominance of cognitivist models and what he terms a 'neo-pragmatist' approach, in favour of an account that considers both social influence and embodied subjectivity in its understanding of mental distress.

CONSTELLATION AND CRITIQUE

The purpose of this volume, then, is to collect an array of different voices, which, when taken together, can illuminate the subject of the interface between mental distress, mental health and the humanities, without offering any programmatic or dogmatic methodology or declaration of intent. The German philosopher Theodor Adorno articulates a form of philosophical critique that is encapsulated in the concept of a constellation of concepts, a constellation that will function as a loose grouping that can be picked out to figure an image of a collective whole, without violating the complexity and contradictions of the material at hand. He writes that:

> As a constellation, theoretical thought circles the concept it would like to unseal, hoping that it may fly open like the lock of a well-guarded safe-deposit box: in response, not to a single key or a single number, but to a combination of numbers. (Adorno, 1966: 163)

This is an apt metaphor for the process of understanding that is at the heart of this book. However, a number of key themes emerge from the collection of voices contained within this volume.

First, the process of understanding that which is, in some sense, beyond understanding is central to the task of any hermeneutic within mental health care. This does not mean that there is a radical split between normality and pathology, or that there is not a continuum of mental states that can cross from the so-called normal to the insane. It means that we should try and think both continuity and discontinuity when trying to understand madness. What does this paradoxical statement mean? I think it means that there are shared aspects of our humanity and ways of being that can figure the difference involved in madness, but also there is a radical discontinuity in some states of what we term madness. Feelings of not being a unified person, not feeling alive, not feeling connected to one's body or to other people have a relation to certain so-called normal experiences, but also in madness they have an intensity that can move them into a realm beyond straightforward understanding. Thus arises the problem of the ineffability of certain mental states and their representation. In extreme states of madness, the person is trying to give voice to something that is inexpressible. This does not mean, though, that it is without meaning. However, the meaning to be deciphered calls for a hermeneutic approach that is as attentive to silences and gaps in meaning as it is to any straightforward narrative or diagnostic picture. Therefore, an ethics of psychiatry arises through this practice of continually trying and failing to understand mental distress both in its continuity with 'normal' experience and in its radical discontinuity from such experience.

Second, this understanding needs to be linked to the wider society and culture within which it takes place. Mental distress needs to be comprehended as a form of life that arises within a societal and cultural context, and that draws attention to the way that our lives are mediated at a deep level by the structures of a society. This is not as a supplement to a biological or a psychological approach, but deeply embedded in any idea of what it means to live our lives as embodied subjectivities within a particular form of the social reproduction of life.

Finally, an account of critical practice in psychiatry needs to be aware of its own complicity with vested interests and power structures and reflect upon its own models and structures to better provide a mental health service that is truly both critical and helpful.

REFERENCES

Adorno, TW (1966) *Negative Dialectics* (EB Ashton, Trans). London: Routledge.

Bracken, P & Thomas, P (2005) *Postpsychiatry. Mental health in a postmodern world.* Oxford: Oxford University Press.

Foucault, M (1995) Madness and the absence of work. *Critical Inquiry, 21,* (2), 290–8.

Jaspers, K (Ed) (1997) *General Psychopathology* (2 vols) (J Hoenig & MW Hamilton, Trans). Baltimore, MD: Johns Hopkins University Press.

McHugh, P (1997) Foreword. In K Jaspers (Ed) *General Psychopathology* (pp v–xii). Baltimore, MD: Johns Hopkins University Press.

Chapter 1

FEELINGS, BELIEFS AND BEING HUMAN

John Cromby

Over the next few days, Jenny slowly lost her hold on reality. The heavy sedative effects [of psychiatric drugs] were accompanied by a restlessness that kept her constantly on the move up and down the ward, muttering under her breath and occasionally pulling up her nightdress to show the nurses her supposedly too-large hips. From time to time she had outbursts ... she threw food and plates around, tried to escape from the ward, swore at the doctors, slammed doors, and hurled herself to the floor ... At other times, it seemed as though her previous worries were all appearing in a distorted form. For instance, she told the staff that Prince Charming had spoken to her from the television ... that she was a film star, and then that she was pregnant. Once she asked anxiously if she had killed her family, and then told one of the doctors 'I'm only three years old'. (Johnstone, 2001: 69)

INTRODUCTION

This chapter describes something of what it might mean to take feelings as the raw stuff of being human. In the first half of the chapter feelings are defined and their status in our experience is described. Their socialisation is then explained, as are some aspects of their relationship to language, and this leads on to a brief consideration of the relationship between feelings and beliefs. In the second half of the chapter the possible relevance of all this for the HUMAN project is then explained with reference to Jenny's story, part of which appears above.

FEELINGS

Primordially, before anything else, being human means being a feeling body. Our experience of the world is delivered up, in all its fantastical immediacy, by a species-nature that bequeaths us, during our waking hours, a ceaseless flow of sensory, haptic, proprioceptive and kinaesthetic signs. This flux, simultaneously both rhythmic and indeterminate, is the originary stuff of experience and subjectivity, and continuously provides the non-representational 'background' (as Shotter, 2003, puts it) from which all formal meaning is condensed. It is not simply that our feeling bodies are in the world, but—as Merleau-Ponty (1962/2002) puts it—our bodies *give* us the world. It is because of our bodies that there is a world for us at all, and so feedback from our bodily senses, capacities, practices, habits, modes of comportment and ways of being continuously contributes to the meanings that constitute our lived, subjective experience.

At its most basic this feedback consists of feelings, elements of experience reflective of the momentary state of our body-brain system as it mediates and enables the situated, relational flow of our being-in-the-world. These feelings flow continuously one into the other, with only the occasional intrusion (e.g. unexpected sharp pain) to interrupt their otherwise relatively seamless flux of somatic textures, affordances, valences, durations and intensities. Feelings are not only central to the entirety of our experience; they also continuously provide our default mode of engagement with the world. The pre-reflective orientation to the world that our feelings supply is the mode of engagement and assessment to which we always return, and upon which we most frequently rely to 'show' us where we are, what is going on, and how we should orient ourselves with respect to it all. Feelings of love, for example, suffuse the entire perceptual world of those experiencing them, and this occurs non-deliberately, before any reflection upon its novelty and beneficence. Feelings, then, are not simply information: although they can be taken as information when we interpret them, we do not have to engage in interpretation for them to have their influence. Indeed, feelings continuously supply the pre-reflective ground upon which all interpretation occurs, functioning to shape and constrain the range of interpretations that it will seem legitimate to make.

Despite their centrality and importance, feelings (with the obvious exception of acute states) frequently avoid our attention. Unless there is something out of the ordinary or wrong, the felt body tends to recede into the background, typically becoming 'the darkness in the theatre needed to show up the performance' (Merleau-Ponty, 2002: 115). Most feelings are relatively vague and metamorphose gradually one into the other, and all are intrinsically non-representational in character: consequently, the majority come and go without being remarked upon or recorded (Langer, 1967). In any case, it is frequently advantageous and adaptive to focus more upon what is happening outside of our bodies than what is happening within them (not least because what is happening within our bodies already influences how we experience what occurs outside of them).

Experientially, then, the felt body is somewhat ineffable, constituting an absent presence that also inflects our formal structures of knowledge. For example, social constructionist and other psychologies have been accused of 'ocularcentrism', an unwarranted prioritisation of the visual sense and concomitant neglect of embodied, practical ways of knowing (Sampson, 1998). Similarly, Western knowledge more generally has been characterised as logocentric, overly concerned with the binary logic of the sign, and with representation (Derrida, 1974).

Although they are experienced continuously and relatively seamlessly, feelings can nevertheless be characterised as falling into one of three groups. First, there are emotional feelings, the corporeal, felt component of emotional states: the involuntary gasp of fear or surprise, the somatic decompression and lightness of joy, and so on. Emotions are relatively complex phenomena, bound up with elements of knowledge, narrative, intention and morality, all of these associated with each other in relationally and societally normative ways. Emotional feelings, though, consist only of the somatic element of these complex hybrids, and in that sense at least are considerably simpler phenomena.

Second, there are extra-emotional feelings: hunger, pain, sexual desire, being tired and so on. This terminology acknowledges that these feelings also have emotional connotations: hunger, for example, is closely bound up with (sub)culturally specific emotional norms, as the lives of people with eating disorders demonstrate (Meyer, Waller & Waters, 1998). In some accounts this class of feelings is dismissed as mere sensation, a dismissal that may in fact mark the point where ocularcentrism and logocentrism are first instantiated. Aside from its epistemic aspects this dismissal is also an implicitly politicised one, since it echoes the association of the so-called 'contact senses' (touch, taste) with both lower forms of life and inferior positions within social hierarchies of class, gender and race. The so-called higher or 'distance senses', by contrast, are associated with rationality (for example in the form of 'vision' or 'insight') and with social positions presumed (at least by some who occupy them) to be 'superior' (Blackman, 2005). Rather than dismiss these feelings as sensation, here they are explicitly recognised as factors that load our experience with valences and textures: hunger endows food with significance and interest, tiredness drains interest and makes effort more difficult, and so on.

Third, there are feelings of knowing, the kinds of feeling characterised in everyday life as intuition or 'gut' feeling, and indexed in conversation with such phrases as 'I just felt there was something else going on'. This class of feelings, whose somatic properties are typically vague, were discussed at length by William James (1892); more recently they have attracted the attention of scholars as diverse as philosopher Susan Langer (1967), neuroscientist Antonio Damasio (1994) and cultural theorist Raymond Williams (1968). In psychology, their most insightful advocate has been John Shotter (1993) who characterises them as 'knowing of the third kind'. Shotter's appellation captures what is most palpable about these feelings, which is that they are intentional and informational. The knowledge they yield is sensuous, 'practical-moral' knowledge, intrinsically bound up with both the ebb and flow of social relations and with the discursively organised and legitimated structures of formal knowledge which we more readily recognise.

Although for analytical purposes feelings can be pre-emptively characterised in these ways, in our lived experience such characterisations are typically post hoc. The subtle, continuous, pre-reflective, non-representational character of our feelings means that deliberate effort is often needed if we are to name them. Moreover, feelings are sometimes contradictory, mixed or shifting, and we frequently have good reason to disavow how we feel (to shield or nurture others, cope with challenging circumstances, or protect ourselves against painful realisations). Consequently, it is usually only once a feeling has become sufficiently intense or enduring, or otherwise had its influence marked for us, that the reflexive act of interpreting and conferring formal meaning upon it is made. Such reflexive interpretations involve the deployment of discursive or other conventionalised, societally obtained resources (e.g. musical notation) and so constitute a route by which our individual embodied experience is socialised. But there is a further sense in which embodied experience is socialised, because the feelings to which we apply these reflexive interpretations are also themselves already socialised.

Drawing upon the three-fold classification presented above, it should be apparent that feelings of knowing are already intrinsically social. On the one hand they are already thoroughly bound up with or called out by our immediate, situated, relational engagements, where they provide us with an ongoing sense of how our relations with others are actually proceeding. On the other hand, they are aligned with wider sociocultural structures and stratifications, most obviously through the ways that modes of comportment and structures of taste, preference and desire reflect societal hierarchies and positions (Bourdieu, 1977). Feelings of knowing may also be understood (if only retrospectively) as reflective of shared, historically emergent sensibilities, not yet capable of being wholly represented by existing social and discursive forms (Williams, 1968).

Emotional feelings, too, are socialised, and this holds even if we imagine that they are produced by relatively asocial 'basic emotion' systems of the kind proposed by Ekman (1992). Basic emotion theories such as Ekman's require us to accept the existence of biologically hardwired 'modules' or 'affect programs', and to this extent seem to greatly circumscribe social influence. However, not only does Ekman concede the existence of other emotions that are socialised (and in some cases even culture specific), he also acknowledges that the 'display rules' (which regulate how and when all emotions should be expressed or performed) are socioculturally derived. But if we consider, for example, the difference between laughter freely released and laughter suppressed, we realise that the expression of an emotion contributes intrinsically and significantly to the feeling of it. So with respect to their feeling dimension, display rules and emotions (whether considered as basic or otherwise) do not in fact remain separate. Over time, the 'display rule' comes to be part of how the emotion is actually felt, an ontogenetic process that blurs any biological encapsulation of the kind presumed by basic emotion theories (Cromby, 2007).

Finally, extra-emotional feelings are also socialised. Taking pain as an example, martial artists, boxers, wrestlers and others subject themselves to training routines that have the effect of gradually raising the threshold beyond which various kinds of pain become unbearable. Through repeatedly hitting objects and people, and through being hit, practitioners of these arts gradually change the ways and the extent to which they experience pain. Practices of sadomasochism similarly involve the gradual enculturation of pain, in search of more intense sexual experiences (Weille, 2002). More mundanely, children's experience of their own pain routinely gets socialised, largely as a consequence of the ways in which parents and significant others respond when they fall over or scrape themselves.

So not only is the flux of felt experience somewhat ineffable, inherently non-representational, and sometimes contradictory, mixed or variable; also, by the time we are able to turn around and reflect upon it, the stuff we are reflecting upon is already socialised, imbued with degrees of somatic sensitivity that mark our current social and material position. This turning around and reflecting involves the deployment of 'metacognitive' resources derived initially from our previous social relations. These resources, most obviously in the form of 'inner speech', are in fact fragments of prior conversation that have been taken up and rendered speechless, and in the process truncated and stripped of predicates (Vygotsky, 1962, 1978). So what often appears to be a most singular and private aspect of our own experience is already social and relational—both in its origin, and in its continuous orientation to aspects of our immediate situation. Thus, both the feelings we reflect upon, and the tools by which we conduct this reflection, have an intrinsically social character.

At this point, it must be emphasised again that those aspects of experience frequently dismissed as mere sensation are also meaningful. Ruthrof (1997) argues at length that bodily feedback provides signs that operate in dynamic, interpenetrative corroboration with other, more formally conceived and conventionally understood sign systems (such as those of language) and so contribute significantly to meaning making. Consequently, the normativity of our reflexive interpreting does not derive only from social convention and cultural practice. The specific ways in which we are able to viably and legitimately interpret our feelings (and indeed the ease with which we can do this in any given circumstance) also depends to some extent upon the particular characteristics of the feeling(s) concerned. Whilst pain is indeed socialised, intense pain nevertheless seems to have some relatively stable phenomenological characteristics: a somatic character that makes it ever-present in our attention and causes a shrinking of attention, a smaller world, a shedding of other concerns, perhaps even a disintegration of personhood (Leder, 1990; Scarry, 1985). However, it is not that intense pain is purely constant, since even at the extremes it can be experienced and reacted to differentially: mountaineer Joe Simpson's account of his determined escape from the dangerous slopes of Siula Grande, despite shattering his leg in a fall, dramatically demonstrates the extent to which even intense pain can be variably experienced (Simpson, 1997). Degrees of phenomenological stability, then, need not imply a separate realm of the purely biological; rather, they indicate the end of a continuum where socialised influence might taper away but still contributes. Such relatively stable characteristics nevertheless starkly illustrate how the lived body continuously influences the meanings we make by virtue of its felt character, as well as by virtue of the socioculturally derived meanings we attach to those feelings.

Thus, our being human is most fundamentally co-constituted from socialised feelings and from the socioculturally normative and relationally prompted interpretations we place upon them. Through acts of reflection conducted in inner speech, conversation or both, we 'fix' or 'cut' the flow of socialised feelings, according to understandings carried in discursive or other social practices. This fixing is pre-reflectively influenced by the very feelings to which it applies, and may in turn, in the lived moment when it occurs, modify the feelings that prompted it by enabling them to be taken as an object of reflection. There is a ceaseless flux of fluid movement between feeling and interpretation, a continuous melding of one into the other, a smooth dialectic of flow and exchange, realisation and suppression, such that feelings can easily come to stand for or take the place of inner speech, and vice versa (Cromby, 2007).

Given all this we should not wonder that our experience is always somewhat opaque to us, for at its centre lie continuously remade social and relational influences, many of them non-representational in character, prompted or interpellated by aspects of the world to which we may fail to consciously attend, and largely enabled by neural mechanisms that operate outside of conscious awareness (Damasio, 1999). So the kind of subjectivity implied by this prioritisation of feelings is an immanent, emergent one that lacks thorough insight, a subjectivity that is pre-reflectively social in both content and process and thus not rigidly bounded or singular. But at the same time, and contra those post-structuralist positions that seem to imply boundless multiplicity (Glass, 1993), the default character of our feelings can also confer some stability. For, whilst many feelings are purely relational, others are dynamically reflective of the enculturated, habitual rhythms of the body, the spatio-temporal features of its location, the diurnal and seasonal rhythms of the environment, and the synaesthetically predictable (Merleau-Ponty, 2002) textures of objects and surfaces. These materially and somatically derived feelings provide degrees of coherence that are 'automatically' sensed rather than worked up through interpretation or reflection. They root us in a specific place in the material world, and in a particular body that is (usually) much the same body as yesterday's—and they do this at the very same time as they are interpenetrated by other feelings that open us up to dynamic, shifting patterns of social and relational influence.

BELIEFS

What this highlights is that our default relationship to our feelings, derived from the continuous embodied engagements we have with the social and material world, is typically one of more-or-less unquestioning faith (Baerveldt & Voestermans, 2005). Our 'automatic' felt or sensed orientation to the world tends to provide the unquestioned (and frequently unnoticed) ground from which we assess and respond to it, and with which our assessments and responses are thereby pre-reflectively inflected. In contemporary psychology these pre-reflective stances are typically called 'beliefs' or 'schema', a terminology that moves them into the ambit of cognitive psychology and allows them to be misunderstood as primarily informational (or alternatively, discursive) in character. By contrast, it follows from the arguments laid out previously that what psychology calls a 'belief' is in fact more properly understood as a socially derived feeling state, allied to a normative matrix of discursive articulations and social practices. The beliefs that cognitive psychology typically presumes to be nodes or decision-points within informational flow charts are most fundamentally feeling states, and they frequently evade accurate reflection and concise articulation precisely because of their largely non-representational, pre-reflective, somatic character. It is from this understanding that the relevance of this way of thinking to the HUMAN project's concern with mental health and distress will now be demonstrated, by exploring some of its implications for the kind of 'delusional' beliefs stated by Jenny in the excerpt that began this chapter.

Johnstone (2001: 65–70) describes Jenny's life history and circumstances, showing how they contained a combination of emotional sensitivity, overwrought family dynamics and conflict, which culminated in a fraught situation that was resolved by Jenny's diagnosis of schizophrenia. The short excerpt that opened this chapter describes Jenny in the days immediately following her diagnosis and hospitalisation, and details some of the beliefs she proclaimed at this time. Johnstone's account sensitively renders these seemingly bizarre beliefs sensible, clearly showing how they relate directly to her social and material circumstances; unfortunately, only a very brief summary is possible here.

Jenny grew up with an ineffectual, distant father and an over-protective, possessive mother; her parents' relationship had irretrievably broken down many years before but its appearance was stonily and ungenerously maintained because of social conventions. At school Jenny had always struggled to make friends, and when she went to college her difficulties continued—compounded now by tentative, barely articulable sexual desires coupled with a self-perception that she was unattractive because she had big hips and freckles. After a lengthy period of sullen withdrawal, social isolation, and much arguing with her parents, with the friendly encouragement of a sympathetic GP Jenny began to make small, determined efforts to gain independence and maybe realise her fantasy of becoming a film star: she began to contact old friends, to go out more, and to diet. But these attempts to develop a life outside the home only produced more anxiety and conflict within it, as they provoked her mother's fears that Jenny would move away and, in so doing, expose the emptiness of her own life and the sham of her marriage. And so the seething tension in Jenny's home erupted into furious conflict, with Jenny screaming that her mother wanted to keep her like a child and her mother screaming back that she was mad and needed to be locked up. A locum doctor called out by Jenny's mother felt unable to resolve the arguing, but was alarmed by Jenny's unusual remarks ('I can fly out of here any time I want, you know … I know the GP is really married to me, I know everything') and so called a psychiatrist and duty social worker. As a result of their assessment, a provisional diagnosis of schizophrenia was made and Jenny was hospitalised.

Johnstone uses Jenny's story to illustrate the causal role of conflictual family dynamics in distress, suggesting that these conflicts are frequently resolved by artificially locating the problem solely within one family member and diagnosing her or him as 'ill'. Here, I want to use Jenny's story in a parallel fashion, to emphasise the role of feelings in both constituting distress and producing unusual beliefs. Strong feelings of various kinds run all through Jenny's story. The home was 'tense', and Jenny's mother continually expressed 'bitterness and resentment' toward her father. When Jenny first became 'withdrawn' and the GP was called out, he decided she was 'confused' and 'unhappy'. Jenny blamed her parents for having created an atmosphere that would 'make anyone miserable', although her optimistic ambition to become a film star nevertheless gave her 'hope'. The GP's support initially triggered positive changes for Jenny, who began going out more even though she found the thought of sex and relationships 'terrifying' and disclosed 'bitter' memories of being teased and ridiculed. One day Jenny came to the surgery alone, unusually 'cheerful and confident', having spent some of her savings on clothes and planned a night out. But the next day the GP received a 'frantic' call from Jenny's mother, saying that Jenny was going mad; he reassured her that this was highly unlikely but as these calls continued he visited Jenny's home a day later. He found Jenny 'openly angry', 'furious' with her mother, who was 'yelling back' at Jenny and calling her crazy. The GP tried to calm the situation but feelings were 'running too high', so he retreated. Some hours later when the locum arrived in his place Jenny was 'extremely agitated', and her mother still 'yelling'. The two had a 'furious screaming match', after which the locum called for psychiatric assistance. After being diagnosed Jenny struggled 'desperately' and on admission to the ward 'angrily' refused to be examined so was forcibly sedated.

Johnstone (2001: 73–4) suggests that whilst most people sometimes speak in metaphors, people in the extremes of distress 'take the process a stage further and start living their metaphors instead' and that this is what psychiatry takes to be their 'delusional beliefs'. Her account clearly shows how Jenny's superficially bizarre beliefs are in fact sensible in the context of her circumstances. It also accords with the notion that beliefs, most fundamentally, are socially derived feeling states, since each of Jenny's beliefs can be related to one or more of the conflicting feelings that came to dominate her life in the days before and after her hospitalisation. For example, Jenny's claim that 'I'm only three years old' might relate to her longstanding feelings of helplessness and disempowerment: in relation to her mother and father, in her inability to change her life for the better, and in the hospital ward where she was forcibly detained. Other beliefs (being pregnant, having killed her family) are imbued with fear and anxiety, relating to Jenny's 'terror' about sexual relations and her reasonable anxiety that, however the current crisis is resolved, her family will never be the same again. More poignantly, Jenny's beliefs that 'Prince Charming' had spoken to her and that she would one day be a film star reflect her thwarted desires to escape the miserable, tense family home and make a better life.

So the understanding of belief as an amalgam of socialised feeling and discourse is consonant with Jenny's story; however, we can also use it to further extend our understanding of her situation by considering in more detail what actually happens in this move from metaphor ('I feel like a little child') to belief ('I'm only three years old'). If beliefs are, most fundamentally, socialised feelings states, such a move must speak to the sheer intensity, depth and persistence of Jenny's feelings of helplessness. Similarly, the unconventional way these feelings inflect her discourse—such that her beliefs are readily taken as delusional—suggests something of their uncontrollability, the way in which Jenny's feelings of helplessness are so powerful and readily present that their unbidden influence might surge forth at any time. I have argued elsewhere (Cromby & Harper, in press) that the key to understanding such intense, uncontrollable feelings is to recognise that they have frequently co-occurred with other strong feelings. Drawing on Scheff (2003) (who in turn draws on the empirical work of Lewis, 1971), Dave Harper and I proposed that feeling traps—mixtures of feelings held in place by relational and other influences—are what may constitute 'florid' states and give rise to 'delusional beliefs'.

Feeling traps arise when strong feelings co-occur and their simultaneous presence causes them to intensify, sustain and generalise each other. They are produced when persistent relational, social and material circumstances effectively 'lock' individuals into complex mixtures of potent feelings; for Jenny these feelings included resentment, frustration, bitterness, sexual desire, affection, helplessness, anxiety, fear, anger and hope. Johnstone highlights something of the complexity of these mixtures of feeling by observing that, whilst Jenny's mother feared Jenny leaving, Jenny herself was frightened to leave even though she desperately wanted to do so. Jenny feared abandonment at the same time as she yearned to be independent; felt angry at her parents at the same time as she needed their love; felt helpless, even as she seethed with anger and resentment. Other aspects of Jenny's behaviour (her shyness, her overly critical stance towards her own body, throwing herself to the floor of the ward) suggest that she also experienced feelings of shame, insecurity, perhaps even self-loathing, feelings that contributed further to the complex affective dynamics of her situation.

Enmeshment within feeling traps can, over time, lead individuals to adopt habits of feeling and ways of relating that already presuppose particular feelingful responses from others. But reciprocally, these ways of relating may only serve to further intensify the various feelings they presume: not only will this further sustain, intensify and generalise them, it will also make further unhelpful relational dynamics more likely. Feeling traps, are inherently relational; Johnstone's account shows that Jenny's mother, too, was gripped by mixtures of powerful feelings, that both reinforced and complemented those her daughter was experiencing. When feeling traps get sufficiently prolonged, they may eventually induce such highly aroused states that self-reinforcing mixtures of feeling surge forth in unpredictable ways. This seems to be what happened for Jenny, whose enduring mixtures of conflicting feelings, locked into place by her actual position of relative social and material powerlessness, became so intense and unpredictable that, even before her hospitalisation, they began driving her discourse in unconventional ways ('I can fly out of here any time I want. I know the GP is really married to me …'). Her diagnosis and subsequent hospitalisation, far from alleviating these powerful feelings, not only intensified them but added further feelings of shock and fear. Consequently, far from abating, Jenny's complex mixtures of extreme feelings began shaping her perceptions to the extent that she heard 'Prince Charming' speaking to her from the television.

It is at this kind of point, where people see and hear things that are not part of the consensual reality of others, that the idea of distress as biological dysfunction or illness might seem to have its strongest pull. Hallucinations are often clearly dysfunctional, outside of 'normal' perceptual experience, and frequently distressing to those who experience them; attributing them to organic dysfunction therefore appears plausible. However, the focus on socialised feelings and feeling traps yields a different explanation, because we already recognise that in everyday life feelings have a continuous influence upon perception. Consider the rose-coloured spectacles of people newly in love, or the flat, colourless world of the deeply miserable. These descriptions are more than mere figures of speech, they are also lay recognitions that the felt, dynamic body helps to generate the world we experience, that—as Merleau-Ponty (2002) argued—the Cartesian split between subject and object is erroneous. Feelings continually inhabit our perceptions: they predispose us to perceive some things rather than others, to attend to some things more than others, and to interpret what we see in particular ways. So it is that people who have lost a loved one frequently 'see' her or him in the faces of passers-by, and people expecting a baby 'see' pregnant women everywhere. Similarly, experimental evidence demonstrates that poor people 'see' high value bank notes as larger (Bruner & Goodman, 1947), people afraid of spiders see them in an array more readily than other people (Ohman, Flykt & Esteves, 2001), and people with eating disorders 'see' their own bodies as larger than they actually are (Jansen, Smeets, Martijn & Nederkoorn, 2006). And in Jenny's case, perhaps, her anguished desires for freedom reached such a pitch that they temporarily overwhelmed the somatically and materially produced feelings that rooted her in the shared consensual world, so that she 'heard' Prince Charming speaking directly to her from the television.

CONCLUSION

The understanding that socialised feelings are our default mode of engagement with the world, coupled with a reconceptualisation of beliefs ('delusional' or otherwise) as amalgams of embodied feeling states and discursive articulations, may yield numerous advantages; there is space here to briefly mention just three.

First, this perspective illuminates both sociological analyses (e.g. Mirowsky & Ross, 1983; Ross, Mirowsky & Pribesh, 2001) and the extensive evidence from psychiatric epidemiology (e,g. Harrison, Gunnell, Glazebrook, Page & Kwiecinski, 2001; Melzer, Fryers & Jenkins, 2004; Ritsher, Warner, Johnson & Dohrenwend, 2001) showing that adverse social and material conditions cause distress. Neither sociology nor psychiatry has provided adequate explanations for these associations; sociology because the subjective realm is not within its province, psychiatry because (largely blind to the sheer complexity, intricacy and force of social influence) it clings to the notion that when only some people exposed to 'the same' adverse conditions experience distress, this is because they are rendered vulnerable by underlying organic diatheses. By contrast, the focus on socialised feelings, inculcated by relational and material influences, allows these causal associations to be theorised more adequately (see Cromby & Harper, 2007).

Second, this perspective helps explain why psychiatric medication can sometimes make a helpful difference, because it works by directly influencing the mixtures of feeling that constitute distress. For example, serotonin-specific reuptake inhibitors (SSRIs) increase the available levels of serotonin in the brain: in this they are functionally similar to the recreational drug ecstasy (MDMA) but their action is somewhat different (subtler, and more prolonged). As Moncrieff and Cohen (2005) propose, SSRIs and other psychiatric drugs induce their own 'abnormal' brain states that may, in some circumstances, be functional. The artificial lightness of mood that SSRIs can induce is beneficial for some people experiencing profound misery, offering them a brief, chemically induced holiday from the worst of their distress. For those with the resources, such respite can even foster insights into how to change their future social and material circumstances for the better. When this happens it can look like there has been a 'cure' but there has been no such thing, not least because there never was an 'illness' in the first place. SSRIs, just as surely as recreational MDMA, are simply inducing feelings (and hence perceptions) that would not otherwise be present; just like those induced by recreational drugs, these feelings and perceptions can sometimes be socially functional (Shedler & Block, 1990), and sometimes not.

Third, the focus on feelings reminds us that there is a profound sense in which states of distress are inculcated and lived through and in the body. This does not mean that we must naïvely treat body as somehow separate from mind, nor indeed as simply reducible to it. Rather, it means that we must recognise the intimate dependence of subjectivity upon the socialised body, which not only enables but also continuously inhabits and informs it. And because this body is always already a body in a social and material world, then the ways that social and material influence impinge upon us and are related to distress must also gain renewed significance. It urges us towards a social materialist perspective (Smail, 2005), from which the enduring maleficent effects of inequality, discrimination, and adverse power relations must gain a renewed significance.

REFERENCES

Baerveldt, C & Voestermans, P (2005) Culture, emotion and the normative structure of reality. *Theory and Psychology*, 15 (4), 449–74.

Blackman, L (2005) The dialogical self, flexibility and the cultural production of psychopathology. *Theory and Psychology*, 15 (5), 183–206.

Bourdieu, P (1977) *Outline of a Theory of Practice*. Cambridge: Cambridge University Press.

Bruner, J & Goodman, CC (1947) Value and need as organising factors in perception. *Journal of Abnormal and Social Psychology*, 42, 33–44.

Cromby, J (2007) Toward a psychology of feeling. *International Journal of Critical Psychology*, 21, 94–118.

Cromby, J & Harper, D (in press) Paranoia: a social account. *Theory and Psychology*.

Damasio, AR (1994) *Descartes' Error: Emotion, reason and the human brain*. London: Picador.

Damasio, AR (1999) *The Feeling of What Happens: Body, emotion and the making of consciousness*. London: Heinemann.

Derrida, J (1974) *Of Grammatology* (GC Spivak, Trans). Baltimore, MD: Johns Hopkins University Press.

Ekman, P (1992) Are there basic emotions? *Psychological Review*, 99 (3), 550–3.

Glass, JM (1993) Multiplicity, identity and the horrors of selfhood: Failures in the postmodern position. *Political Psychology*, 14 (2), 255–78.

Harrison, G, Gunnell, D, Glazebrook, C, Page, K & Kwiecinski, R (2001) Association between schizophrenia and social inequality at birth: Case-control study. *British Journal of Psychiatry*, 179, 346–50.

James, W (1892) The stream of consciousness, from *Psychology*. Retrieved 25th January 2006 from <http://psychclassics.yorku.ca/James/jimmy11.htm>.

Jansen, A, Smeets, T, Martijn, C & Nederkoorn, C (2006) I see what you see: The lack of a self-serving body-image bias in eating disorders. *British Journal of Clinical Psychology*, 45, 123–35.

Johnstone, L (2001) *Users and Abusers of Psychiatry* (2nd edn). Hove: Brunner-Routledge.

Langer, S (1967) *Mind: An essay on human feeling (Vol 1)*. Baltimore, MD: Johns Hopkins University Press.
Leder, D (1990) *The Absent Body*. Chicago: University of Chicago Press.
Lewis, HB (1971) *Shame and Guilt in Neurosis*. New York: International Universities Press.
Melzer, D, Fryers, T & Jenkins, R (2004) *Social Inequalities and the Distribution of the Common Mental Disorders*. Hove: Psychology Press.
Merleau-Ponty, M (2002) *Phenomenology of Perception*. London: Routledge. (Original work published 1962.)
Meyer, C, Waller, G & Waters, A (1998) Emotional states and bulimic psychopathology. In H Hock, J Treasure & M Katzman (Eds) *Neurobiology in the Treatment of Nervous Disorders* (pp 271–89). London: Wiley.
Mirowsky, J & Ross, CE (1983) Paranoia and the structure of powerlessness. *American Sociological Review, 48*, 228–39.
Moncrieff, J & Cohen, D (2005) Rethinking models of psychotropic drug action. *Psychotherapy and Psychosomatics, 74*, 145–53.
Ohman, A, Flykt, A & Esteves, F (2001) Emotion drives attention: Detecting the snake in the grass. *Journal of Experimental Psychology: General, 130* (3), 466–78.
Ritsher, JEB, Warner, V, Johnson, JG & Dohrenwend, BP (2001) Inter-generational longitudinal study of social class and depression: A test of social causation and social selection models. *British Journal of Psychiatry, 178* (suppl 40), s84–s90.
Ross, CE, Mirowsky, J & Pribesh, S (2001) Powerlessness and the amplification of threat: Neighbourhood disadvantage, disorder and mistrust. *American Sociological Review, 66*, 568–91.
Ruthrof, H (1997) *Semantics and the Body*. Toronto: University of Toronto Press.
Sampson, EE (1998) Life as an embodied art: The second stage—Beyond constructionism. In BM Bayer & J Shotter (Eds) *Reconstructing the Psychological Subject: Bodies, practices and technologies* (pp 21–32). London: Sage.
Scarry, E (1985) *The Body in Pain*. Oxford: Oxford University Press.
Scheff, T (2003) Male emotions/relations and violence: A case study. *Human Relations, 56* (6), 727–49.
Shedler, J & Block, J (1990) Adolescent drug use and psychological health: A longitudinal inquiry. *American Psychologist, 45*, 612–30.
Shotter, J (1993) *Conversational Realities: Constructing life through language*. London: Sage.
Shotter, J (2003) 'Real Presences.' Meaning as living movement in a participatory world. *Theory and Psychology, 13* (4), 435–68.
Simpson, J (1997) *Touching the Void*. London: Vintage.
Smail, DJ (2005) *Power, Interest and Psychology: Elements of a social materialist understanding of distress*. Ross-on-Wye: PCCS Books.
Vygotsky, LS (1962) *Thought and Language* (E Hanfmann & G Vakar, Trans). Cambridge, MA: MIT Press.
Vygotsky, LS (1978) *Mind in Society: The development of higher psychological processes*. Cambridge, MA: Harvard University Press.
Weille, KL (2002) The psychodynamics of consensual sadomasochistic and dominant-submissive sexual games. *Studies in Gender and Sexuality, 3*, 131–60.
Williams, R (1968) *Drama from Ibsen to Brecht*. London: Chatto & Windus.

CHAPTER 2

TOWARDS A CRITICAL PERSPECTIVE ON 'NARRATIVE LOSS' IN SCHIZOPHRENIA

PHILIP THOMAS

Tired of all who come with words, words but no language
I went to the snow-covered island.
The wild does not have words.
The unwritten pages spread themselves out in all directions!
I come across the marks of roe-deer's hooves in the snow.
Language but no words.
From March 1979, Tomas Tranströmer

INTRODUCTION

Tomas Tranströmer's beautiful poem reminds us how texts dominate our lives. Words seduce us into believing that the only way in which we can become fully human is through narrative. Tranströmer shows us that meaning exists in the absence of words, a point that is worth remembering when we consider the growth of interest in narrative across the humanities and the human sciences over the last 50 years. In medicine it is argued that we may think of illness in terms of narratives that are located within the wider narratives of people's lives; adopting a narrative approach to illness is more holistic, and tackles its existential significance (Greenhalgh & Hurwitz, 1999). Narrative also serves the important ethical purpose of helping clinicians and patients to understand more clearly what sort of help the patient needs (Heath, 2001). Narrative is increasingly important in psychiatry, for example in psychotherapy (Holmes, 2000) and rehabilitation (Roberts, 2000), as well as primary care (Launer, 1999). There is, however, another side to narrative in psychiatry. With the exception of Glenn Roberts' work it tends to exclude people with the most severe psychoses such as schizophrenia.[1] This point is rarely made

---

1. Throughout this chapter I will use words like schizophrenia and recovery, particularly where they have been used by other writers. In using these words it must not be assumed that I am accepting them at face value, as though they are straightforward and unproblematic. The main purpose of this chapter is to propose a critical perspective on the relationship between narrative and psychosis. The most appropriate context in which to explore this is schizophrenia, because some particularly interesting work has been written about this.

explicit; it is, however, implicit in Jaspers' assertion that in psychiatry there are limits to understanding, particularly in schizophrenia (Jaspers, 1963). Despite this, throughout history many people who have experienced madness have been moved to write their own narratives. Gail Hornstein (2007) has compiled a bibliography of over 600 First Person Narratives (FPNs) of madness, the earliest being that of Margery Kempe who wrote an account of her madness in the early fifteenth century. Although these narratives have not been subject to detailed study, it seems likely that many were written by people who would probably be diagnosed today as suffering from schizophrenia. Personal stories about the experiences of madness have been a persistent and significant feature of human life throughout history.

Narrative is also central to contemporary debates about psychosis for another reason. There is a strong argument that narrative, and narrative processes, play a key role in recovery from psychosis (Roe & Davidson, 2005; Bracken & Thomas, 2005). For the survivor movement, recovery involves speaking out, the act of reclaiming language, or, as Coleman (1999) has put it, having a voice. Without a language, a voice to speak with, and an audience to hear what is to be said, there can be no story and no recovery. Through social action the survivor movement has created safe, or 'ethical' spaces (Blackman, 2001) in which individuals can begin the process of sharing their stories (Crossley & Crossley, 2001). Yet at the same time there is a paradox here, for the dominant view is that schizophrenia is such a severe condition, one that leads to such a profound loss of selfhood, that the possibilities of narrative and recovery through narrative are generally considered implausible.

There is a powerful tension here. Whilst it is arguable that narrative offers a useful way of thinking about illness and recovery, especially the social and cultural processes that lie at the heart of whatever recovery is,[2] there is a very strong tradition in psychiatry that holds that schizophrenia is debarred from recovery. The cultural tropes that constitute schizophrenia are those of deterioration and deficit (Barrett, 1996), and, ultimately, the annihilation of the self. I will start this chapter by examining those clinical features of schizophrenia that are arguably most closely related to narrative or narrative failure, so-called thought disorder. How are we to interpret silence, or the absence of narrative that appears to be a feature of psychosis? Does silence mean that the person has lost narrative? Does losing narrative mean that you are annihilated and cease to exist as a person? Is it possible to remain a person if you lose narrative? I will argue that a critical exploration of these issues in relation to the condition known as schizophrenia raises serious questions about the relationship between narrative and personhood, both in relation to madness, and more generally in terms of subjectivity and identity. It also opens up the possibility of new and ethical ways of thinking about narrative in psychosis. The noun 'schizophrenia' is laden with meanings that shape our actions towards those who carry the label. In the introduction to *History of Madness* Foucault writes:

---

2. An excellent example of this is the philosopher Susan Brison's (2002) powerful book *Aftermath*, in which she describes the role of narrative in reconstructing the self following trauma, through her personal experiences of recovering from a murderous sexual assault.

> There is no common language: or rather, it no longer exists; the constitution of madness as mental illness, at the end of the eighteenth century, bears witness to a rupture in dialogue, gives the separation as already enacted, and expels from the memory all those imperfect words, of no fixed syntax, spoken falteringly, in which the exchange between madness and reason was carried out. The language of psychiatry, which is a monologue by reason *about* madness, could only have come into existence in such a silence. (Foucault, 2006: xxviii)

Ultimately any attempt to understand the narrative loss of those diagnosed 'schizophrenic' would do well to consider the role that psychiatry, under the influence of its own cultural and historical assumptions, plays in this silence.

SCHIZOPHRENIA, PSYCHOPATHOLOGY AND NARRATIVE

Foucault's insight into the silencing of madness is a penetrating insight, all the more so because he casts it in linguistic terms '... imperfect words, of no fixed syntax ...'. Narrative takes many forms and has many meanings, but the sense in which I use the word here relates specifically to stories in texts and words, and our ability to use texts and words as tools to convey the meaning of our lives by sharing stories about ourselves. In this light there is nothing new in the idea that schizophrenia is linked to difficulties in narrative; the association can be traced back to the origins of the concept. For Bleuler (1911/1950), thought disorder (TD) was a key symptom of schizophrenia. 'Loosening of associations', a disturbance in thought processes, was one of four primary features of the condition, along with changes in affect, and autism (or withdrawal from reality). For much of the twentieth century TD was regarded as a key symptom of schizophrenia, although in recent years interest in the phenomenon has waned.[3]

In recent years the renaissance of scientific psychiatry, what has come to be called neo-Kraepelinism, was marked by the publication of two papers. Klerman (1978) set out a manifesto for a new scientific psychiatry, with the emphasis on description of 'symptoms' in attempts to improve the classification of psychiatric disorders. In a paper titled *The Dementia of Dementia Praecox*, Johnstone and colleagues (1978) invoked the spirit of Kraepelin by drawing attention to the idea that schizophrenia is a condition with poor outcome, leading to 'deterioration' in intellectual and social function, and the 'defect state' so characteristic of those who tragically found themselves dwelling on the back wards of the old asylums. This had many consequences. The notion of 'deterioration' and 'defect state' gave credence to the idea that loss of self occurs in schizophrenia. For example, writing in her book *The Broken Brain,* Nancy Andreasen (1984) described the disease process in schizophrenia leaving behind the empty shell of the person. Disturbances in the experience of selfhood is implied by this extract from DSM-III:

---

3. This is partly because of difficulties in defining it reliably and partly because of the growth of interest in language and narrative (Thomas & Fraser, 1994; Thomas, 1995).

> [T]he sense of self that gives the normal person a feeling of individuality, uniqueness and self-direction is frequently disturbed in schizophrenia. (APA, 1980: 189)

Neo-Kraepelinism emphasised the importance of scientific rigour and conceptual neutrality. It attached particular importance to clarity in symptom definition and description as a means of overcoming the notoriously low inter-rater reliability of psychiatric symptoms. One consequence of this was the emergence of interest in the distinction between positive and negative symptoms of schizophrenia (Crow, 1980). Positive symptoms include unusual experiences, such as hearing voices, and unusual beliefs, that are not present in 'ordinary' people.[4] In broad terms, they correspond to the symptoms of acute psychosis. Negative symptoms, on the other hand, are more difficult to define and identify reliably, because they represent 'deficits', or a reduction in or loss of a previously 'normal' capacity. However, they correspond closely with the 'defect' state traditionally associated with chronic schizophrenia. The distinction between positive and negative symptoms pertains across the full range of the subjective experience in psychosis, including language and communication, mood, cognition and perception, but I want to focus on the distinction as it relates to disturbances in language and communication.

In her work on the Thought, Language and Communication Scale (TLC), Nancy Andreasen (1979a, b) makes no a priori assumptions about the nature of thought disorder (TD), and instead provides detailed descriptions of abnormalities of verbal behaviour commonly observed in interviews between psychiatrists and their patients. Some time ago I examined the TLC and demonstrated that its constituent items could be accounted for in linguistic terms (Thomas, 1995). For example, Andreasen's definition of incoherence and fragmentation (examples of so-called positive thought disorder) correspond closely in linguistic terms to disturbances of syntactic (sentence) structure. Derailment (positive thought disorder) and loss of goal[5] are both disturbances that occur at the level of the text. Interestingly, in linguistic terms the majority of Andreasen's items may be seen as failures of pragmatics. These include poverty of speech and poverty of content of speech (both varieties of negative thought disorder), as well as pressure of speech, distractible speech and tangentiality (varieties of positive thought disorder). In terms of narrative, however, disturbances of the structure of texts and pragmatics[6] have implications for how a person's narrative integrity is likely to be judged by a listener. So,

---
4. There is of course abundant evidence that this is not so, and that psychotic experiences such as hearing voices or unusual beliefs are to be found relatively commonly in the public at large.
5. The position of loss of goal is ambiguous. In some ways it may be seen as a positive symptom, perhaps as a loss of narrative coherence, but equally it may be seen as a consequence of the negative symptom, poverty of content of speech.
6. Again in broad terms, we may think of anything more than one sentence in length as a text. This is to distinguish between linguistic approaches that are primarily concerned with the sentence level, for example syntax and transformational grammars, from those that are concerned primarily with the meaning of larger bodies of texts, such as narrative. Pragmatics, on the other hand, is primarily concerned with how speakers use language to convey meaning in social contexts. Pragmatic disruptions are particularly likely to impede a speaker's ability to narrate his or her story in the presence of a listener.

returning to the positive-negative dichotomy, we can see that positive thought disorders are broadly characterised by incoherent narratives, in which the listener's ability to understand, interpret and make sense of the speaker's utterance is compromised. Under such circumstances, listeners are likely to conclude that narrative intelligibility is impaired. It is worth recalling that in chapter two of *The Divided Self*, Laing (1965) sets out the importance of understanding and hermeneutics in relation to madness, drawing on Dilthey's analogy concerning the interpretation of human action with the interpretation of hieroglyphics and other ancient texts. Laing makes a direct comparison between the interpretation of ancient hieroglyphs and the interpretation of 'psychotic "hieroglyphic" speech and actions' (Laing, 1965: 31).

Negative thought disorders, on the other hand, are characterised by a *pragmatic* failure, that of generating insufficient speech (or narrative) or in its most extreme form, silence, a failure to generate *any* speech or narrative. To make the point more clearly, let us consider Andreasen's definitions of poverty of speech and poverty of content of speech. Poverty of speech involves a 'restriction in the amount of spontaneous speech' (Andreasen, 1982). Replies to questions are brief and unelaborated, or may be monosyllabic. In severe cases there may be little or no spontaneous speech, and the person may be mute. Poverty of content of speech is defined as a pattern of speech which whilst adequate in amount, conveys little in the way of information. In mild forms it is characterised by repetitious speech full of pause fillers and false starts. In more severe forms it is characterised as empty philosophising. The point here is that negative symptoms, particularly poverty of speech, appear to correspond closely to the loss of narrative and self that has recently been described in psychosis.

SCHIZOPHRENIA AND NARRATIVE LOSS: SILENT SELVES?

At this point I intend to explore the relationship between narrative loss and schizophrenia as it has recently been conceptualised by psychiatrists who have an interest in philosophy and psychopathology. For the sake of simplicity I will focus on negative symptoms and narrative loss. This is not to imply that narrative loss does not occur in people who show evidence of positive thought disorder. But the problem here is slightly different. It is, as Laing suggested, one of interpretation and the reconstruction of meaning from what might be regarded as a fractured narrative. This is a major undertaking beyond the scope of this chapter, although it is worth noting in passing that attempts have been made to reconstruct the meaning of disordered narratives, in schizophrenia (Hydén, 1995) and autism (Gray, 2001). Roe and Davidson (2005) have also shown how the reconstruction of narrative is a central feature of recovery from schizophrenia. Here, my purpose is a critical examination of the claims that have been made about loss of narrative in schizophrenia, particularly in relation to the presence of negative symptoms of schizophrenia.

The intersection of psychopathology and philosophy at the locus of schizophrenia and narrative is important because of the claims that are made about selfhood in psychosis. A themed edition of the journal *Philosophy, Psychiatry and Psychology* under the title

Agency, Narrative and Self examined amongst other things the issue of narrative loss in psychiatric disorders. The issue began with a series of case vignettes (Wells, 2003), one of which described the case of 'Joanne', a young woman who first presented to psychiatrists at the age of 16 with a six-month history of loss of motivation and direction. She said to her psychiatrist, 'I'm gone'. A diagnosis of schizophrenia was made, and over the next six years she developed marked affective blunting, to the extent that her emotional responses were 'almost non-existent' (Wells, 2003). Commenting on Joanne's case, Phillips (2003) points out that six years later Joanne's narrative self had all but disappeared. He makes this judgement on the basis of the clinical finding of the negative symptom of affective blunting:

> As indicated, the fact that her emotional response is 'markedly blunted, almost non-existent at 22' suggests that the narrator who was present at 16 is now gone. In contrast to the poignant, rich narrative we heard at 16, we now hear none at all or one that is flattened out, concrete, devoid of emotion, and rather stereotyped. (Phillips, 2003: 322)

The first point to make here is that Phillips' argument about loss of self is established on the basis of Joanne's blunting of affect. He does not refer particularly to poverty of speech. However, the nature of negative symptoms, at least as far as the internal consistency of rating scales such as Andreasen's 'Schedule for the Assessment of Negative Symptoms' is concerned, is such that blunting of affect and poverty of speech are highly correlated with each other. Joanne's downward course leading to 'deterioration', blunting of affect and negative symptoms, in other words the emergence of the 'defect state', leads Phillips to suggest that in schizophrenia the narrator may fade to a point where it makes 'decreasing sense to speak of a narrative self' (ibid: 323). The appearance of the 'defect state' means that the subject vanishes.

Phillips suggests that Joanne presents us with a paradox when she declares 'I'm gone'. The question is who is this 'I' that has gone, but at the same time is capable of declaring its own departure. Originally she declared:

> Where I was is filled with noise and voices, and there's—it's a small area, the brain, but there's a huge emptiness there that I used to fill. (Wells, 2003: 299)

Despite the empty spaces and poignant absences we still hear a narrative 'I', but six years later this narrative self has all but disappeared. Again, Phillips makes this judgement on the basis of the clinical finding of affective blunting:

> What remains, perhaps, is a self that is emotionally blunted, tied to the concrete details of her ongoing life, and who has *lost her capacity for reflective (or prereflective) reaching into the past or future*. It is an impoverished self and one that in diminishing degrees qualifies as a narrative self. (Phillips, 2003: 319-20, emphasis added)

I want particularly to draw attention to the idea that Phillips introduces here, that the self has the capacity to reflect, and in doing so, reach back into the past or forward into the future. This idea attaches particular importance to the continuity of the relationship between self at different points in time. The capacity to be aware of self at different points in time is, in Phillips' view, part of our capacity to be reflective, and that the loss of this capacity, which is associated with the presence of negative symptoms, impoverishes selfhood, and in particular the extent to which one qualifies as a narrative self. The downward course of Joanne's condition has resulted in Joanne the narrator fading away to a point where it makes 'decreasing sense to speak of a narrative self' (ibid: 323). There are two issues that Phillips' paper raises, and which I want to consider in detail. The first arises from the way in which clinicians decide whether or not a person shows evidence of blunting of affect or poverty of speech. Blunting of affect is assessed on the basis of a reduction in emotional expressivity, for example reduced facial expressiveness, prosodic qualities of speech and a reduction in the use of expressive hand gestures whilst speaking (Andreasen, 1982). Given that the assessment of poverty of speech is based on the presence of a 'restriction in the amount of spontaneous speech' (Andreasen, 1979a), doesn't this presuppose some notion of what normal amounts of speech production should be? In other words this is an evaluation that presupposes narrative normativity. Indeed, is it possible to take this further and question the view that personhood should be attributed solely on the basis of the amount and quality of speech that we appear capable of generating, or for that matter the amount of emotional expressiveness we evince when we speak? Second, in the presence of a silent other with a diagnosis of schizophrenia, how can we be certain that the silence that we experience reflects narrative loss, or the loss of the self of the person who remains silent? Are there other ways in which we might understand silence?

In general terms, loss of narrative is regarded as a fixed and enduring feature of people who are diagnosed as suffering from schizophrenia. Not everyone agrees. Such a pessimistic view stands in marked contrast to the more hopeful position taken by Roe and Davidson (2005), and leaves no space for subtle shifts and changes in the extent to which a person may evince narrative at different times, and in different contexts. Narrative loss may be temporary; Clive Baldwin (2005) points out that people may lose and regain narrative agency. So, perhaps not all selves are narrative selves all the time.

The focus in Phillips' paper is on the narrative, rather than the person and the contexts in which the narrative is situated. He removes narrative from the embodied and historical contexts which make narrative possible in the first place. In doing so, he elevates the status of narrativity, holding it up as the sole determinant of what it means to be a human being. This is not to say that narrative is unimportant in human identity, but I want to question the emphasis that Phillips places on narrative and its relationship to selfhood. To assume that Joanne's silence is to be understood in terms of her narrative loss is to overlook the possibility that contextual factors influence the extent to which Joanne feels she can, or wants, to be a narrative being. But she remains a person. This indicates a danger of narrative. The importance we attach to narrative in understanding selfhood paradoxically limits the possibilities of becoming for those whose narrative fails to conform to certain norms. I want now to explore this by questioning the idea that it is only through narrative we manifest selfhood.

IS NARRATIVE A NECESSITY FOR SELFHOOD?

Narrative plays an important role in recent philosophical theories about the nature of selfhood. Phillips (2003) draws attention to the work of four philosophers whose work has helped to shape the view that narrative is central to selfhood. The most important figure behind the ideas of philosophers like Alasdair MacIntyre (1981), Paul Ricoeur (1984) and David Carr (1986) is Martin Heidegger (1962). His insight that human being is fundamentally historical opens up the possibility of thinking of human lives in narrative terms. The argument here is that if human being is fundamentally temporal in nature, then it must be experienced narratively. Like a good story, a human life must have a beginning, a middle, and an end, and have a good plot. This does not mean that the finished text is the narrative. Philosophers like MacIntyre who advocate for narrative identity argue that we live narrative tentatively, contingently, reflexively and pre-reflectively. The important point here is that it's not the completed narrative that's important. In reality our narratives are only finished when we die, and even then others may continue to write and re-write our stories. What is important is the struggle to impose, or at least to attempt to impose, narrative order on inchoate and emergent experience. MacIntyre (1981) argues that human action is only intelligible insofar as it is embedded in a historical sequence. Thus narrative, meaning, human action and history are interrelated.

Galen Strawson's (2004) polemically titled essay, *Against Narrativity*, questions the extent to which we should think of ourselves as inevitably narrative beings. He presents a cogent critique of the narrative trend in disciplines such as philosophy, psychology, medicine and anthropology. He begins by proposing that the argument that human subjectivity may be thought of in narrative terms can be divided into two related theses, psychological Narrativity and ethical Narrativity.[7] The former is an empirical view of how human beings experience their lives. The latter is a normative, or moral, thesis which maintains that to experience our subjectivity in narrative terms is desirable because a richly narrative subjectivity is a prerequisite for a good life. In general terms the view that dominates many is that both theses are true; human beings are fundamentally narrative beings, and that to be so is necessary if we are to lead good lives. Strawson contests this:

> It's just not true that there is only one good way for human beings to experience their being in time. There are deeply non-narrative people and there are good ways to live that are deeply non-narrative. (Strawson, 2004: 429)

---

7. He capitalises 'Narrativity' here in order to 'denote a specifically psychological property or outlook' (Strawson, 2004: 428).

To insist upon the truth of both theses closes down important areas of thought, impoverishes our ethical possibilities, hinders our understanding of ourselves, and, most important of all, 'needlessly and wrongly distress[es] those who do not fit their model' (ibid: 29).

Strawson would probably broadly agree with Phillips on the importance of temporality in relation to subjectivity and narrative, but he would almost certainly reach quite different conclusions about the significance of the relationship. Phillips argues from a Heideggerian perspective, that we may consider the relationship between narrator and narrative to be one that is deeply rooted in the historicity of human being. The narrator is in the present, relating what has happened in the past, or at least an account of past events, together with an account of possible future events. This is precisely how he describes the failure of Joanne's narrative on pages 319–20 of his paper. A narrator narrates from within the perspective of his or her own present, describing how psychopathology influences the expression of historicity within the narrative. But in chronic schizophrenia characterised by deterioration:

> [I]t barely makes sense to speak of historicity. The patient exists in a stagnant present that barely should be called a present, because it is so minimally related to a past and a future. (Ibid: 324)

This is a restricted and limited reading of the significance of temporality in relation to being-in-the-world. Phillips' view implies that our experience of temporality is linear, the Newtonian arrow from past through present into future, from which as subjects we stand outside, disengaged, observing, dipping in and out at will. For Heidegger, temporality is *constitutive* of being. There is no linear time frame, and the present is constantly engaging and disengaging with different time frames in our lives. It is not atemporal, detached and outside time as Phillips seems to suggest (Bracken & Thomas, 2005). Strawson argues that those like Phillips who advocate for 'narrative' subjectivity overlook the complexity of our relationship with time. He distinguishes between two fundamentally different forms of human relatedness to time, the diachronic and the episodic. In the former, upon which the claim for both narrativity theses is based, we hold a clear view of how we were in the past and the continuity of this view through the present into the future. In the latter we have no enduring sense of the continuity of ourselves over time. Strawson suggests that these differences are fundamental, and that an individual's position on the episodic–diachronic continuum may vary, for example depending on our state of health. He writes:

> [W]hen I am experiencing or apprehending myself as a self ... the remoter past or future in question is not my past or future, although it is certainly the past or future of GS [author] the human being. (Strawson, 2004: 433)

Most significant here is his view that there are important moral and ethical implications that arise from the distinction between episodic and diachronic:

> I'm well aware that my past is mine in so far as I am a human being, and I fully accept that there's a sense in which it has a special relevance to me*[8] now, including special emotional and moral relevance. At the same time I have no sense that I* was there in the past, and think it obvious that I* was not there, as a matter of metaphysical fact. (Ibid: 434)

Strawson is heavily critical of the ethical narrativity thesis—that narrativity is necessary for the good life, and he questions this with reference to his own life. He points out that it is perfectly possible to have a firm notion of oneself as a person, and to live a good life without being concerned about questions such as 'What has GS made of his life?', which beg to be answered in ethical narrative terms:

> This does not mean that I am in any way irresponsible. It is just that what I care about, in so far as I care about myself and my life, is just how I am now. The way I am now is profoundly shaped by my past, but it is only the present shaping consequences of the past that matter, not the past as such. (Ibid: 438)

In other words, we may be perfectly able to act as moral beings without being diachronic, that is to say without an enduring sense of continuity from past to present, without narrative. He concludes that both ethical and psychological Narrativity theses are false.

Woody (2004) also draws attention to the problems that arise if we insist that narrative is a necessity for selfhood. If the self is nothing more than the invention of narrative then we run into the danger of reducing subjectivity to text. Foucault (1979) warned about this in the *History of Sexuality*, where he argued that there was no deep 'innermost' subjectivity accessible through psychotherapy. Attempts to locate identity in narrative risk detaching the self from its own experience. It is impossible to be engaged with experience if we talk about it. Experience is immediate, embodied and situated. A story cannot tell itself; stories require narrators. But stories must also be rooted in the narrator's experience, so Woody reformulates the question of narrative loss in psychosis by asking whether the phenomenon is an aspect of the experience of psychosis rather than narrative failure as such:

> Perhaps the narrative failure is only a symptom that reflects or represents a fragmentary experience that thwarts narrative integration. (Woody, 2004: 333)

This is important in the context of Strawson's work. Our predilection for thinking of self and identity in terms of narrative tied to text and language is problematic for those episodic individuals in whom narrative may not play such an important role. Woody's argument raises another possibility, that so-called narrative loss in psychosis may arise through the failure of words to articulate experience. Brendan Stone (2004) makes a similar point in a series of papers on narrative, selfhood and schizophrenia. Likewise the novelist Sarah Maitland (2007) has written about the inadequacy of words to convey

---

8. The use of 'me*' and 'I*' is Strawson's way of distinguishing between self-referential statements within specific phenomenological contexts.

anything about those aspects of our lives that relate to mystical states, spiritual or sexual rapture, and psychosis. Taken together, this suggests that rather than simply accepting silence as a fact indicative of an absence of self, we must adopt a more sophisticated approach to silence, one that implies that we may need to consider other ways of expressing our selfhood beyond, or without, words.

Phillips' view that the silence of schizophrenia indicates the loss of self is firmly rooted in both the descriptive (psychological) and normative (ethical) narrativity theses. It assumes that human lives are to be expressed in narrative terms, and that it is necessary to be a narrative being in order to have a life that is worthy and good. This is clearly based in a value judgement about the importance of narrative in our lives. Being a person ultimately depends on our ability or willingness to express ourselves discursively, in ways that conform to a particular view of what narrative is. Those who do not conform to these norms are said to have lost narrativity. But the problem isn't simply that of thinking of selfhood in narrative terms, but thinking that the only possible way to evince narrative is through words. Woody points out that it is one thing to find words to describe intense emotional states such as grief or love, but a completely different thing altogether to tell stories about them. In our attempts to express such powerful, ineffable states, we turn to poetry and music, forms of expression that either stretch the limits of words, or forego word-based language altogether. Secondary discursive processes and verbal thought dominate psychology to the exclusion of other forms of thought such as imagery and fantasy. This insistence on the primacy of language troubles Woody:

> I have no doubt that some people do assemble themselves by telling themselves stories about themselves ... For some, the image, the melody, the dance are more congenial and eloquent means of expressing and formulating experience than language. (Ibid: 335)

CAN SILENCE HAVE MEANING?

At this point I want to consider some empirical evidence that supports the conceptual arguments developed here, and challenges the view that silence in schizophrenia indicates loss of self. There is good evidence that although people with chronic schizophrenia may be silent, they have neither lost narratives nor their selves. Corin and Lauzon (1992) describe a single case study using interview and other data from 'Mr. A', a socially withdrawn man with a ten-year history of schizophrenia and high levels of negative symptoms. He is described as very withdrawn from the world, with few friends and low work expectations. His daily activities were very limited and ritualised, for example visiting parks, cheap restaurants, walking inner-city streets, taking trips on buses. Their interview data shed light on his withdrawal, which he framed in a meaningful way. He fully recognised that he was an uncommunicative person, but he understood this in terms of his deep antipathy towards a society which in his view was lacking in love and compassion. His withdrawal or 'negative symptoms' emerge as deeply meaningful in the context of his critical perspective on a harsh world. His withdrawal served as a retreat, a place to go when he required 'peace and quiet, or when he wants to escape the mess created by his father in the rest of the house' (Corin & Lauzon, 1992: 273). There he would meditate, listening to the 'vibration of silence'. Meditation changed the value of his withdrawal, justifying it, imbuing it with meaning and purpose. Religious signifiers were an important aspect of this. His closeness to God improved how he felt about himself:

> It is not an ideal society for giving a sense of security to the person who is sick. The hardest is society itself, the way of life it tries to impose upon us. They only think of production, and judge us according to it ... Society will never get me to change my mind about what is most valuable: It is not money but God, the inside.[9] (Mr. A, in Corin & Lauzon, 1992: 274)

Objectively, Mr. A's life may have appeared empty, characterised by 'deficits' and 'dysfunction'. However, he saw his withdrawal as a way of reconstructing his personal relationship with the world in a rich and meaningful way. In contrast to the empty self implied by clinical descriptions, Mr. A's self is not only present and intact, but imbued with spirituality.

Bouricius (1989) describes the discrepancies between objective assessments of her son's negative symptoms and the emotional richness of his inner world as reflected in his writings over many years. Ratings by seven people (including psychiatrists, her own and her son's self-ratings) of his negative symptoms indicated that he had moderately severe poverty of speech. Her concern is that people with negative symptoms may be misunderstood because they have difficulty in expressing their thoughts through words, and feelings through facial expression and gesture. Her son's writing, much of it in the form of poetry, reveals a rich and complex emotional world, as well as an acute awareness of his difficulties in communicating with others:

> Stuck in my thinking, brain
>   paralyzed between fear and
>   love.
> Stuck on you. Stuck between
>   the last word and the next.
> Stuck by confusion, the
>   inability to proceed any fur-
>   ther in understanding or
>   speech.
> Oh well, I'm just stuck again.
> (Bouricius, 1989: 205)

---

9. Perhaps one way of interpreting Mr. A's comment here is that unbeknownst to him he is following the philosophy of St. Augustine. Taylor (1989) points out that it was Augustine who proposed that we should look inside ourselves to discover truth, because that is where we will discover God. Augustine places the emphasis on the activity of knowing (or epistemology) in contrast to the world of objects, because knowing is inner and that is where God is.

And:

> Went to see my doctor, but couldn't talk. Kept saying, 'I don't know,' to his questions. Started crying. Felt pity and love for Rhoda because she has fear, because she has to take medication, because she is a mental patient like me, because I want to marry her, but I think I never can. I started saying that I had lost my memory. Then I got up and left.
> (Bouricius, 1989: 206)

These extracts show that objective assessments of negative symptoms simply fail to convey the richness of subjective experience. It is a serious error to assume that silence and lack of emotional expression signal the loss of self in schizophrenia. In other circumstances we are perfectly happy to accept that such features serve a purpose and have meaning. A professional card player depends on not divulging any information about his or her reactions to a deal by maintaining an unchanging facial expression despite being highly aroused. We speak of someone being 'poker-faced'. A person suffering from severe myasthenia gravis may have a complete lack of facial expressiveness, but can still experience deep emotions. We recognise that as part of their spiritual devotion, members of some religious orders, such as the Order of Cistercians of the Strict Observance (Trappists), observe strict silence in their lives.

CONCLUSIONS

What has been described as narrative loss in schizophrenia is, as Clive Baldwin notes (2005), primarily an ethical issue. An important implication of his paper is that whilst it may be the case that psychosis compromises our ability to produce narrative, this places us under an obligation not to assume that this is so. The case that I have argued here supports his view. It is not enough for us to dismiss narrative silence as evidence that the person has lost selfhood. It is wrong to do so for two reasons. It presupposes that narrative is a necessity for selfhood. In addition, empirical evidence suggests that even in the presence of severe negative symptoms, those clinical features most likely to lead to the judgement that someone demonstrates narrative loss, a richly narrative self may remain. This is why Baldwin's point about the ethics of narrative in psychosis is so important. 'Narrative loss' places us under an obligation to search for the person, and at the same time, question our own assumptions about the nature of narrative and its relationship to the self. Woody (2004) proposes that we should move away from the hegemony of language to other forms of narrative expression, such as dance, music, and performance, to which I would add poetry (which has the power to twist and distort words and texts into new meaning) and the visual image. This is exactly what some survivors of mental health services have been doing for many years. In *Dedication to the Seven*, Louise Pembroke (2007) uses dance to tell the story of her relationship with her voices. Aidan Shingler (2007) uses images to tell his story about the way that he was silenced *not* by his madness, but by psychiatry. These powerful and inspirational stories conveyed in a language without words challenge our conception of narrative, and in doing so, what it means to be human.

REFERENCES

American Psychiatric Association (1980) *Diagnostic and Statistical Manual of Mental Disorders* (3rd edn). Washington, DC: APA.

Andreasen, N (1979a) Thought, language and communication disorders: I: Clinical assessment, definition of terms, and evaluation of their reliability. *Archives of General Psychiatry, 35*, 1315–21.

Andreasen, N (1979b) Thought, language and communication disorders: II: Diagnostic significance. *Archives of General Psychiatry, 36*, 1325–30.

Andreasen, N (1982) Negative symptoms in schizophrenia: Definition and reliability. *Archives of General Psychiatry, 39*, 784–8.

Andreasen, N (1984) *The Broken Brain: The biological revolution in psychiatry*. New York: Harper & Row.

Baldwin, C (2005) Narrative, ethics and people with severe mental illness. *Australian and New Zealand Journal of Psychiatry, 39*, 1022–9.

Barrett, R (1996) *The Psychiatric Team and the Social Definition of Schizophrenia*. Cambridge: Cambridge University Press.

Blackman, L (2001) *Hearing Voices: Embodiment and experience*. London: Free Association Books.

Bleuler, E (1950) *Dementia Praecox or the Group of Schizophrenics* (J Zinkin, Trans, 1950). New York: International Universities Press. (Original work published 1911.)

Bouricius, J (1989) Negative symptoms and emotions in schizophrenia. *Schizophrenia Bulletin, 15*, 201–8.

Bracken, P & Thomas, P (2005) *Postpsychiatry: Mental health in a postmodern world*. Oxford: Oxford University Press.

Brison, S (2002) *Aftermath: Violence and the remaking of the self*. Princeton, NJ: Princeton University Press.

Carr, D (1986) *Time, Narrative, and History*. Bloomington, IN: University of Indiana Press.

Coleman, R (1999) *Recovery: An alien concept*. Gloucester: Handsell Publishing.

Corin, E & Lauzon, G (1992) Positive withdrawal and the quest for meaning: The reconstruction of experience among schizophrenics. *Psychiatry, 55*, 266–78.

Crossley, M & Crossley, N (2001) 'Patient' voices, social movements and the habitus; How psychiatric survivors 'speak out'. *Social Science and Medicine, 52*, 1477–89.

Crow, T (1980) Molecular pathology of schizophrenia: More than one disease process? *British Medical Journal, 280,* 66–8.

Foucault, M (1979) *History of Sexuality Vol 1: An introduction* (R Hurley, Trans). London: Allen Lane.

Foucault, M (2006) *History of Madness and Civilization* (Preface to the 1961 edn) (J Murphy & J Khalfa, Trans). London: Routledge.

Gray, D (2001) Accommodation, resistance and transcendence: Three narratives of autism. *Social Science and Medicine, 53,* 1247–57.

Greenhalgh, T & Hurwitz, B (1999) Narrative based medicine: Why study narrative? *British Medical Journal, 318,* 48–50.

Heath, I (2001) 'A fragment of the explanation': The use and abuse of words. *Journal of Medical Ethics and Medical Humanities, 27,* 64–9.

Heidegger, M (1962) *Being and Time* (J Macquarrie & E Robinson, Trans). Oxford: Basil Blackwell.

Holmes, J (2000) Narrative in psychiatry and psychotherapy: The evidence? *Journal of Medical Ethics and Medical Humanities, 26,* 92–6.

Hornstein, G (2007) *Bibliography of First-Person Narratives of Madness in English* (3rd edn). Accessed 8th November 2007 at <http://www.mtholyoke.edu/acad/assets/Academics/Hornstein_Bibliography.pdf>.

Hydén, L-C (1995) In search of an ending: Narrative reconstruction as a moral quest. *Journal of Narrative and Life History, 5,* 67–84.

Jaspers, K (1963) *General Psychopathology* (J Hoenig & M Hamilton, Trans) (See especially p 305). Manchester: Manchester University Press.

Johnstone, E, Crow, T, Frith, C, Stevens, M, Kreel, L & Husband, J (1978) The dementia of dementia praecox. *Acta Psychiatrica Scandinavica, 57,* 305–24.

Klerman, G (1978) The evolution of a scientific nosology. In J Shershow (Ed) *Schizophrenia: Science and practice* (pp 99–121). Cambridge, MA: Harvard University Press.

Laing, RD (1965) *The Divided Self: An existential study in sanity and madness.* Harmondsworth: Penguin.

Launer, J (1999) A narrative approach to mental health in general practice. *British Medical Journal, 318,* 117–19.

MacIntyre, A (1981) *After Virtue.* Notre Dame, IN: University of Notre Dame Press.

Maitland, S (2007) Effing the Ineffable: Finding a language for prayer, madness and passion. Paper presented at Manchester Cathedral. March, 2007.

Pembroke, L (2007) *Dedication to the Seven* (DVD). Accessed 14 November 2007 at <http://www.intervoiceonline.org/2006/12/19/dedication-to-the-seven-hearing-voices-in-dance>.

Phillips, J (2003) Psychopathology and the narrative self. *Philosophy, Psychiatry and Psychology, 10,* 313–28.

Ricoeur, P (1984) *Time and Narrative Vol 1* (K Mcloughlin & D Pellauer, Trans). Chicago: University of Chicago Press.

Roberts, G (2000) Narrative and severe mental illness: What place do stories have in an evidence-based world? *Advances in Psychiatric Treatment, 6,* 432–41.

Roe, D & Davidson, L (2005) Self and narrative in schizophrenia: Time to author a new story? *Journal of Medical Ethics and Medical Humanities, 31,* 89–94.

Shingler, A (2007) *One in a Hundred.* Accessed 14 November 2007 at <http://www.oneinahundred.co.uk/>.

Stone, B (2004) Towards a writing without power: Notes on the narration of madness. *Auto/Biography, 12,* 16–33.

Strawson, G (2004) Against narrativity. *Ratio, 22,* 428–52.

Taylor, C (1989) *Sources of the Self: The making of the modern identity.* Cambridge: Cambridge University Press.

Thomas, P (1995) Thought disorder or communication disorder: Linguistic science provides a new approach. *British Journal of Psychiatry, 166,* 287–90.

Thomas, P & Fraser, WI (1994) Linguistics, human communication and psychiatry. *British Journal of Psychiatry, 165,* 585–92.

Tranströmer, T (1997) From March 1979. In *New Collected Poems* (R Fulton, Trans) (pp 134–5). Newcastle upon Tyne: Bloodaxe.

Wells, L (2003) Discontinuity in personal narrative: Some perspectives of patients. *Philosophy, Psychiatry and Psychology, 10,* 297–303.

Woody, M (2004) When narrative fails. *Philosophy, Psychiatry and Psychology, 10,* 329–45.

Acknowledgements

Discussions, conversations and arguments with many people have influenced this paper. I am particularly grateful to Clive Baldwin, Gail Horstein, Sara Maitland, Louise Pembroke, Brendan Stone Tim Thornton and Alison Tom for sharing their ideas and thoughts, and in doing so, helping to shape my own ideas and thoughts.

CHAPTER 3

CONSTRUCTIONS, RECONSTRUCTIONS AND DECONSTRUCTIONS OF MENTAL HEALTH

Ian Parker

When we approach the concept of 'mental health' there is, of course, always a question in our minds; what is this 'mental health' that we intend to examine? These two words 'mental health' might, we think, be preferable to the couplet 'mental illness'; but, tempted as we might be to find some neutral terminology to approach this crucial research question, we know as qualitative researchers that every word we use is semiotically loaded, rich with meanings that will always locate words in discourses we may not want to endorse. We may, for example, want to avoid the notion that people who suffer distress are 'ill', but the use of the term 'health' instead of 'illness' does not altogether escape medical discourse. And there still remain the problematic connotations of the term 'mental', for that presupposes that our objects of study are internal psychological states. Contemporary discourse is replete with words and images that locate the causes for our activities inside individual minds; we increasingly inhabit a 'psychological culture' that delimits the horizons of our inquiry (Gordo López, 2000; Parker, 2007); and so the construction, reconstruction and deconstruction of those horizons of what is thinkable are what I am concerned with in this chapter.

I will illustrate my argument with examples designed to evoke what we might call 'mental health' as a cultural practice. That means being specific about the cultural examples, and I will show how this cultural specificity also bears upon the kinds of methodology we use to study mental health. I will take my examples from Finland—with a specific focus on the city of Tampere—and Finnish culture, which does abound with certain specific images of 'mental health', and I will make clear that my exploration of cultural images is conducted from the standpoint of someone working in Manchester—a peculiar post-industrial twin for Tampere.[1] In this way we will produce some 'eurovisual' reference points for 'mental distress'.

METHODOLOGICAL REQUIREMENTS

Whatever 'it'—this 'mental health'—is, it is a cultural practice, and to explore this cultural practice qualitatively there are some key requirements, and these are already methodological requirements.

---

1. A version of this chapter was originally presented at the Qualitative Research on Mental Health Conference, Tampere, Finland, June–July 2006.

PARTICULARITY OF CONTEXT

The first is particularity of context. Cultural practice is always something specific, even in conditions of rapid globalisation that appears to suffocate local traditions. It is necessary to attend to this process of globalisation as always also 'glocalization' in which local particularities of context are shattered and recomposed, deconstructed and reconstructed (Robertson, 1995). One only has to think of the phenomenon of 'world music' to see how local practices are abstracted and repackaged as part of the process of commodification for an international market.

Whatever might emerge as a 'transcultural' field of world mental health, then, will always have to manage the particular ways in which people from different parts of the world are classified and experience peculiar simultaneously normalised and pathologised emotional conditions of life. So, for example, we know that there are historical semiotic links between Tampere and Manchester. There have been some similarities of industrial development, and Tampere is sometimes referred to as the Manchester of the North, or 'Manse'.[2] This is then apparent in the term for a form of Finnish rock music known as 'manserock'.[3]

There are a few Finnish families in Manchester, and until quite recently there was a Finnish-language school. This transcultural aspect of contemporary life even has consequences for what the BBC represents as good mental health. Anna, according to one BBC 'videonations' report, says that 'some of the scenery and buildings of the city centre [in Manchester] remind her of Tampere so much she hardly ever feels homesick'. The report continues 'All she has to do is take a walk around Castlefield with her husband Matti.'[4]

The deep cultural connections between Finnish and English culture are also useful here as an opportunity to draw attention to other cultural components that also connect with specific references to emotional states of well-being and un-ease, if not dis-ease. The Moomins, characters invented by the Finnish author Tove Jansson, first appeared in the London *Evening News* in 1954. I remember as a child being puzzled by the rather strange depressive figures that appeared in the books about Moominvalley.[5] The 'hattifatteners', for example, are rather dangerous beings that travel in groups, with their only apparent goal being to reach the horizon (which is an issue that will also be of relevance for us here). Already, you see, there is cultural differentiation at work around what we imagine mental health to be. There is a permanent Moominvalley exhibition at the Tampere Art Museum, open every day,[6] and there is a museum shop. Everything in the capitalist world can be commodified, including our fantasies and emotions.

You could say that these figures from Moominworld function in some way as

---

2. 'Tampere', <http://en.wikipedia.org/wiki/Tampere> (accessed 7 June 2006).
3. 'Manserock', <http://en.wikipedia.org/wiki/Manserock> (accessed 7 June 2006).
4. Alojoki, A 'Home from home', <http://www.bbc.co.uk/videonation/articles/m/manchester_homefromhome.shtml> (accessed 7 June 2006).
5. See 'Moomin', <http://en.wikipedia.org/wiki/Moomin> (accessed 7 June 2006).
6. 'Tampere Art Museum—Moominvalley', <http://www.tampere.fi/muumi/english/> (accessed 7 June 2006).

representations of emotional states; we are able to attend to them, acknowledge them, but still keep them at a safe distance. The representation of something disturbing to us can actually be comforting if we can perhaps contain it. You will notice here that the way I am framing this relationship to disturbing things is quite therapeutic, and I will reflect on the prevalence of therapeutic discourse later on.

PARTICULARITY OF FOCUS

The second requirement is particularity of focus. Here we must address some problematic issues in qualitative research.

Some versions of discourse analysis focus on the actual things that appear in a text, and will refuse to go beyond that (see, for example, Potter, 1998). So, for example, if 'power' is not spoken about in a text, then it would not be legitimate to speak about power in the analysis. This approach is actually very English, and in line with a longstanding tradition of English empiricism; it is a tradition of research in which only things that can actually be observed are taken seriously. This discursive research is thus a form of 'textual empiricism'. It is quite well suited to a quantitative research paradigm, of course, but it is very problematic when it starts to stipulate what should be spoken about in qualitative research. When we are concerned with issues of mental health it becomes even more problematic.

This is a lesson that we can draw from the work of Michel Foucault, for in his history of madness, he emphasises that his study is about particular kinds of 'dividing practices' that separate reason from madness (Foucault, 2006). His is an account which circumscribes the shape of madness by tracing what reasonable discourse has to say about it. His account is thus formulating a boundary between reason and madness, showing us how something other than reason operates, operates as an empty space, a silence that itself defines what it is we fill with speech.

Some versions of discourse analysis also try to locate themselves within the accepted boundaries of social scientific practice by adhering to quantitative research concerns with sampling and with kinds of 'data' that can claim to be representative. In that kind of research the assumption is that the larger the number of instances there are of a particular phenomenon the more confident we can be that we have found something worthwhile. The problem, however, is not only that a collection of instances drowns out the specificity of a case that is being analysed, but also that this approach prioritises what is 'evident'.

There are more fruitful alternatives to this that are more congruent with the work of Foucault and with the general tenor of deconstructive analyses of cultural forms. Roland Barthes' (1957/1973) classic semiological analysis of the figure of the black soldier saluting the French flag on the cover of *Paris Match*, for example, had to conjure up the network of significations that operate as the condition of possibility for this image. We now recognise from feminist anti-racist work in qualitative research that we need to attend to the way that the pathologised presence of certain representations of a category of subject goes alongside normalised absence of certain representations (Phoenix, 1994). Notice, for example, that we do not actually see the French flag in the text Barthes analyses, and we certainly do not see the whole of the French occupation of

Algeria in this image. It operates, instead, as a 'telling case' that we must decode and locate, deconstruct and reconstruct (see Stanley & Wise, 1983).

What is hidden from view may actually be more important, a more telling case, than what is evident. This is surely the way that ideological practices work to enforce certain kinds of normality and to pathologise certain kinds of experience; to make it invisible. The feminist movement, for example, developed out of activities of 'consciousness-raising' which brought into public discussion a multitude of experiences that had been hidden from view. In that process, what was brought into consciousness was reconstituted; certain conditions of possibility for speaking about experience transformed the experience itself. The speaking subject that emerges is always already positioned in relation to existing dominant categories of subject.[7]

PARTICULARITY OF HISTORY

In addition to these two methodological requirements—particularity of context and particularity of focus—there is a third methodological requirement, which is particularity of history, or, we could say, 'temporal particularity'.

If we turn again to Foucault's work we can see that the careful historical reconstruction of who we have come to be now is only possible because the kinds of questions we ask are questions about how to develop a 'history of the present' (Blackman, 1994). This history is a history of the changing boundaries that divide what is accepted from what has been excluded. So, in qualitative research that draws on Foucault's work, the focus on certain telling cases is a way of exploring a whole domain of discourse, and thus providing an analysis of how that discourse functions to constitute not only what we can immediately see as a number of countable instances, but what we cannot see and what only appear momentarily at certain points (Parker, 2005).

You might imagine that each telling case operates as an item in a projective test. Foucault was actually quite interested in projective tests, and administered Rorschach blot images to patients when he was working as a clinical and forensic psychologist, though this was years before he moved on to write about the history of madness and then genealogies of other concepts (Parker, 1995). Take the set of items from what has come to be a distinctively Finnish projective test, 'Wartegg'.[8] Many people, including students to be selected to study psychology, are given this test in Finland. The subject must doodle in the squares, and what they draw can be analysed; and there are other variables taken into account, which include the order in which they choose to fill in the different squares. Some items are included to make the subject feel anxious; one square with a little black square dot in it was designed to elicit anxiety, and so the interpretation will rest not only on what the subject draws but also how many other items they will prefer to fill in before they turn to tackle that one.

---

7. Finland was the first European country to grant votes to women, in 1906.
8. For a general overview of Wartegg in the context of projective tests see, for example, Cohen de Lara-Kroon (nd) 'The history of projective testing (emphasizing the thematic apperception test', http://www.cohendelara.com/publicaties/history.htm (accessed 19 June 2006). The Wartegg items can be found at <http://www.wsu.edu/~converse/wartegg.html> (accessed 19 June 2006).

There is a crucial difference between a projective test and the analysis of discursive practice however; in our analyses we examine how the categories that are used to produce a definable object that lies within reasonable discourse have been produced and how these categories function. Once again, this is a quite different notion of discourse to that which has become acceptable in the empiricist tradition. Discourse is not a massive observable corpus of statements, but it operates through certain potent signs, words, images which crystallise and speak of what is not spoken everywhere else.

CONCEPTUAL MOVES

We need to make two conceptual moves if we are to develop the qualitative research tradition further in order to tackle representations of mental health.

ATTEND TO THE BOUNDARIES

The first is to direct qualitative research not to 'mental health' as such but to the boundary that divides health from illness, normality from abnormality, reason from unreason. I use a number of oppositions here as if they are synonymous, as if they neatly map onto to each other. Of course they do not. The question that we ask when we attend to the boundary is precisely what it is that is constituted on our side of the boundary—within the discourse we are able to use to speak about it—and what is produced as the disturbing, unsettling, frightening stuff on the other side of the boundary.

However, this kind of inquiry also needs to embed the analysis in relations of power and relations of ideology. The history of 'madness', to use a shorthand term just for a moment, is also a history of other relationships between the powerful and the powerless. The semiotic stuff and material practices that divide reason from unreason have always drawn upon, mobilised and transformed a range of other axes of domination and oppression. Path-breaking though Foucault's work on madness, discipline and confession has been, he did not adequately address the ways that class, culture and sex were always implicated in the construction of what we take to be 'normal' and 'abnormal' (Sawacki, 1991).

To bring those other axes of oppression into the analysis is not to weaken or dilute it, but actually strengthens the analysis we can then provide of the way 'mental health' operates across the fabric of society. Then we can see how mental health operates across the boundaries that simultaneously separate and constitute different categories of subject. One set of discussions around this kind of analysis comes from within feminist research, and around the attempt to conceptualise 'intersectionality' (see, for example, Yuval-Davis, 2006). To rehearse the argument very briefly here; in Western culture, we can see how the intersection between pathology, class, culture and sex has tended to operate.

First, the working class has traditionally been seen as the brutish mass that was insufficiently individuated to be able to engage in sophisticated 'talking cures', and mob behaviour in which the masses had completely taken leave of their senses was feared by psychological theorists. Second, those outside the civilised world were represented in the colonialist imagination and then in orientalist imagery as closer to nature, barbarians who were more likely to be afflicted by a variety of exotic pathological conditions. Third, femininity has historically been associated with madness. One only has to think of the images of 'hysteria' that were contrasted with what people took to be the norm, which was good strong masculine reason.

ATTEND TO BOUNDARY CHANGES

Let us move on to the second conceptual move, which is to attend to how the boundaries change.

This is where I want to turn to specific 'telling cases' to illustrate how some important changes might be operating so we can think about what the consequences might be. I want to tease out boundary changes that have taken place quite recently and the way those boundary changes are necessarily implicated in different axes of domination and oppression beyond 'mental health'.

ANIMALS

A matter of great concern in recent critical work in psychology has been over the way certain kinds of emotions are essentialised. That is, they are turned from culturally specific descriptive terms into things that researchers in the positivist tradition then imagine can be identified in each and every human being whatever culture they inhabit. Critical work on the social construction of emotion has been a very useful corrective to this positivist tradition (Harré, 1986). However, the process of essentialising emotions is not restricted to that tradition of research. The spread of therapeutic discourse in Western culture has actually been a more potent force in encouraging us to think that we can isolate and 'resonate' with certain emotions.

This has also entailed a reformatting of the boundary between human beings and animals, and there is here a new version of the cultural practice of anthropomorphising. Treating animals as endowed with human motivations and emotions is not new in West European culture. There was a time when animals could be tried for various crimes and sentenced in courts of law (Evans, 1906/1987). However, what we are faced with now is something new, for animals can be represented as having emotions which we do not necessarily find threatening—far from it; now we might actually connect with those emotions after they have been distilled into quack remedies.

Incidentally, there was, at the beginning of the twentieth century a sub-speciality of psychology called 'plant psychology'. One study of the psychological index and psychological abstracts uncovered many titles of articles concerned with plant behaviour and even the 'mental life of plants' (Crellin, 1992). Like the criminal trials of animals, such things are wiped away by history because they become unthinkable when new epistemological and ontological boundaries are installed in a culture.

The language of connection and resonance with emotions to describe a practice that will facilitate mental health is an intrinsic part of contemporary therapeutic discourse. This therapeutic ethos relies on the identification and mobilisation of distinct emotional states, and those who refuse to acknowledge and value these states are liable to be treated as pathological in some way; defensive at the very least. Every such specification of mental health entails a specification of how mental pathology will be understood, and it is our task as qualitative researchers to trace how the boundaries between the normal and abnormal are constructed and warranted.

Emotions always cluster around the motif of gender, and alongside the essentialising of emotions in new age therapeutic remedies we find the essentialising of gender itself. However, now something has changed in the boundary between masculinity and femininity. I noted earlier that femininity has historically been associated with madness, and this was certainly the case at the end of the nineteenth century at the time of the birth of modern psychiatry and psychology (Ussher, 1991). Therapeutic discourse, however, requires a view of emotion as something positive, something to be embraced, instead of something to be shut away.

The assumption that it is healthy to be 'emotionally literate' has transformed femininity from being a threat into being an asset (Burman, 2006). And, correlatively, this assumption transforms masculinity from being something eminently reasonable, once privileged over femininity, into something that is now a liability. It is now men who are the problem in Western psychological culture. The boundaries that define mental health have thus changed, and the intersection between these boundaries and other kinds of boundary between different categories of subject, here feminine and masculine, have to be included in our analyses.

SAMURAI

A second telling case is to be found in something more specific, in the motif of the 'samurai sword' in images of madness in British culture. It is not widespread, and it is not discussed endlessly, but it is a sign which condenses a number of different elements that are at play in Western conceptions of reason and what we imagine is 'other' to reason.

I do not know how far this image resonates in other West European countries, but there is something emotionally charged in images of the samurai in Britain. It is part of a more general orientalising of Japanese culture, and Japan functions often as a limit case culturally and in social research; it is simultaneously similar and different (Burman, 2007; Parker, 2008a). The images of the samurai connote a romanticised vision of the warrior, but it is far enough away for it not to function as a threat.

Before I turn to some specific instances where this imagery has been mobilised, it is worth noting that the semiotic linkage between this orientalist image of the warrior and some kind of madness has been present for some years in US American culture, and so it has also already been present to the British public. A classic episode of *Star Trek*, 'The Naked Time' which was first screened in 1966 had the crew of the Enterprise infected by a strange virus that afflicted each one of them in distinctive ways. This narrative device reveals some deeper assumptions about personality traits and what categories of subject are likely to contain them. One of the nurses, for example, bursts into tears and declares her love for Mr Spock.

The key example here, though, is Mr Sulu who starts racing around with a fencing sword. An apparently trivial point, well-known to trekkies, is that the writer of this episode 'originally planned to have Sulu wield a samurai sword, but George Takei [the actor] convinced him that a samurai sword was too "ethnically consistent" for a worldly 23rd-century officer, so it was replaced with a fencing sword'.[9] Here is an issue for semiologists, for we have at play an image that functions by virtue of its chain of associations, and by what was absent rather than by what was present in the image.

In recent years the samurai sword has bubbled into public consciousness in Britain as something associated with madness. Let us turn to some brief examples from recent news reports.

From November 2000, the headline runs 'Man "flipped" in pub attack' and the first line of the story reads 'A Swindon man who brandished a two-foot-long Samurai sword in a Merseyside public house has been placed on probation for two years.'[10] The sword offence is described as 'bizarre' in the story, and the use of the signifier 'flipped' evokes a moment of madness.

From July 2001, 'Swordsman's mother defends son' and the first line of the story reads 'The family of a schizophrenic man shot dead by police as he brandished a Samurai sword have denied he was a danger to the public.'[11] In this case the police in Liverpool were already so certain that someone with a samurai sword was dangerous that he was shot dead.

From June 2002, we now have 'Samurai sword attacker freed' and the first line of the story reads 'A man detained indefinitely after attacking 11 churchgoers with a samurai sword has been released after less than two years, it has emerged.'[12] This story reassures readers that 'Seventy per cent of schizophrenics respond to treatment for their condition and new drugs on the market are far more successful at treating the illness', and so the medical model is evoked to contain the outrage provoked by the story.

From March 2003, a story with the title 'Loud party sparks samurai threat' and the first line of the story reads 'Driven up the wall by the racket from a St Valentine's party, a Spa man threatened his neighbour with a Samurai sword.'[13] The phrase 'driven up the wall' functions here to evoke something of the madness that must have led someone to use a samurai sword.

From September 2003, the headline runs 'Samurai sword killer is sent to mental hospital' and the first line of the story reads 'The samurai sword killer of a hero political aide, who grew up in Daresbury, has been sent to a mental hospital indefinitely—but only a medium security institution.'[14] There is, perhaps, an implication here that it is the use of the samurai sword that demands more than a medium security institution.

From April 2004, 'Teenager admits killing father with Samurai swords' and the first line of story reads 'A teenager has admitted murdering his father by stabbing him

---

9. 'The Naked Time (thing)', <http://everything2.com/e2node/The%2520Naked%2520Time> (accessed 5 June 2006).
10. <http://archive.thisiswiltshire.co.uk/2000/11/23/230910.html> (accessed 5 June 2006).
11. <http://news.bbc.co.uk/1/hi/uk/1441582.stm> (accessed 5 June 2006).
12. <http://news.bbc.co.uk/1/hi/england/2073623.stm> (accessed 5 June 2006).
13. <http://archive.thisisworcestershire.co.uk/2003/3/19/220797.html> (accessed 5 June 2006).
14. <http://archive.thisischeshire.co.uk/2003/9/9/164994.html> (accessed 5 June 2006).

repeatedly with two samurai swords.'[15] In this story the teenager is reported as saying that Satan had told him to carry out the attack.

From October 2005, we read 'Samurai sword used in town attack' and the first line of the story reads 'A man in his 50s has escaped serious injury after being attacked by a man wielding a samurai type sword in County Down, police have said.'[16] Notice here the telling phrase 'samurai type sword'.

From May 2006, the headline runs 'Man killed with samurai sword in drug feud' and the first line of the story reads 'Police are hunting two men after a drug feud ended with the murder of a suspected dealer with a samurai sword.'[17] Here the 'drugs' function as signifiers that serve to explain why such a bizarre thing might happen.

We should note here the reiteration of the link between madness and violence, as if it could be taken for granted that someone who carries out violent acts must be mentally disturbed and as if mental ill health necessarily entails that they will be dangerous. There is a semiotic link here with the 'diagnoses' that are routinely given of political opponents to prove that they are mentally unbalanced and so a threat to Western civilisation (Immelman, 1999, 2003). Once again, you may also notice that we have a string of cases in these newspaper reports of masculinity run riot, and some orientalism mixed in for good measure in the motif of the samurai sword.

ORCS

Let us turn to a third example of what I hope will serve as another telling case.

It was once said that Hell will freeze over before Finland wins the Eurovision Song Contest, and I do remember one contest in which the Finnish contestant Kojo got zero points.[18] One story is that his song 'Nuku Pommiin'—which we could translate as 'sleep to bomb'—refers to sleeping too late. Ironically, on the day when the finals took place, he did indeed sleep too late and missed the contest.[19] One history of Eurovision says that his was 'the worst-rated song in a final'.[20] But on the 20 May 2006, of course, Lordi had a frighteningly triumphant win (with the highest score in Eurovision history). There had supposedly been attempts by Christian groups in Greece, mobilised through an anti-Lordi campaign 'Hellenes', to exclude the band from the country.[21] According to one account, then, Lordi are Satanists.

According to another account they are like the Orcs from Tolkien's *Lord of the Rings*. There has been discussion of this in the English press, including the observation that if the contest was to be held in Mordor there would be a danger that The Shire and

---

15. <http://scotlandtoday.scottishtv.co.uk/content/default.asp?page=s1_1_1&newsid+3344> (accessed 5 June 2006).
16. <http://news.bbc.co.uk/1/hi/northern_ireland/4305068.stm> (accessed 5 June 2006).
17. <http://www.guardian.co.uk/drugs/Story/0,,1777213,00.html> (accessed 5 June 2006).
18. <http://www.yle.fi/eurovision/data/historia.php> (accessed 19 June 2006).
19. I thank Teija Nissinen for this anecdote (personal communication, 19 June 2006).
20. Eurovision Record Book, <http://eurovision.tummiweb.com/main.html?page=voting> (accessed 19 June 2006).
21. It seems now that this 'protest' movement was a publicity stunt designed to work in favour of Lordi.

Rivendell would automatically award each other 12 points (Wroe, 2006). You see the way chains of signifiers operate to link together quite different fields of culture.

The discourse circulating around Lordi is relevant to our discussion here precisely because of the way it marks a distinction between public and private, and between what is a performance on the one hand, and a rational individual subject who lies behind the mask on the other. There has been much speculation about why the band will not take off their masks, so it would seem that there is an absolute identity between the surface 'madness', as we might say, and the rational subject who is merely playing at being demonic. This would give space for psychological notions to be mobilised, and then it would make sense for the lead singer Mr Lordi to say, for example, in an article in the *International Herald Tribune* that 'In Finland we have no Eiffel Tower, few real famous artists, it is freezing cold and we suffer from low self-esteem' (Bilevsky, 2006).

This is a perfect opportunity, then, to recycle stereotypes about Finns, but you should notice here the role of a psychological variable 'low self-esteem', for it is operating as a reassuring buffer-zone concept between us and pure evil, between us normal folk and unmitigated pathology. The coordinates of that formal opposition between the normal and the pathological can then be filled with a rich variety of ideological content depending on the particular context.

We have already explored how axes of gender, race and class become superimposed on the opposition between sanity and madness, but there are always a host of other culturally specific indicators that people have lost their minds. We only have to recall the panic about 'brainwashing' after the Korean War, and the fear that communists might exert some kind of thought control to manipulate people. The 2004 remake of the classic film *The Manchurian Candidate* is symptomatic here: originally made in 1962 but pulled from the cinemas after the Kennedy assassination, the film then starred Lawrence Harvey who was programmed by the Reds to shoot the US president. The mother was a communist agent who triggered the assassination attempt by showing her son an image he had been implanted with, which was the Queen of Diamonds playing card.

The remake of the film, made after the fall of the Berlin Wall, shifted to some vague conspiracy involving oil corporations in the Middle East, and so now the 2004 version is in line with a diffuse sense that big business is pulling the strings. There has been a significant cultural shift from the years of the Cold War, and this shift has consequences for representations of mental health. The coordinates of paranoia are always located in the most potent images of threat.

So, back to Lordi. In one Finnish cartoon a girl is asking her friend 'how will you recognize him?' and the other girl replies, as they turn the corner to meet a frightening Lordi figure, 'he said he will have a flower in his buttonhole' (which he does). The joke here is that Lordi are known to be really nice, sweet people. But the question remains, why don't they take off their masks? There have been rumours in Finland that the band members are KGB agents sent to Finland by Vladimir Putin to destabilise the country and so prepare the way for a Russian-led coup.

However, even this is a rather comforting layer of talk, and it is clearly part of the game, part of the game in which fans collude with a performance knowing it is just that, a performance. For example, after the band won the Eurovision contest there was discussion about what Tomi Putaansuu, the lead singer and former film student, really looked like; but when a magazine (*7 Päivää*) did publish a photograph of Tomi without a mask, and two days later the other four band members were unmasked by another magazine (*Katso!*), a petition signed by over 130,000 people called for a boycott of the magazine in protest (and 130,000 out of a Finnish population of under five million is quite a lot).

The separation between public persona and the real person backstage was confirmed in newspaper reports; for example, in *The Guardian*, the report went like this: 'Scratching his nose with a plastic talon after his band's victory, Mr Lordi said,

> In Finland, they've said things like we eat babies for Christmas. Whenever we appear in public people do their best to ignore us ... We are not Satanists. We are not devil-worshippers. This is entertainment. Underneath [the mask] there's a boring normal guy, who walks the dogs, goes to the supermarket, watches DVDs, eats candies. You really don't want to see him. (Booth & Smith, 2006: 3)

This is the giveaway. You don't want to see him because it would dispel the illusion, but the fact that it is an illusion is exactly what needs to be maintained. An 'illusion' signals that all is well, and there is certainly not a confusion between reason and what lies beyond, no delusion that would indicate that we have tipped into an abnormal realm from which there will be no escape (Parker, 2008b).

CONSTRUCTION ET CETERA

We have examined the construction of some images, but this still leaves some loose threads concerning reconstruction and deconstruction. As the historically constituted boundaries change around different constructions of mental health there is a continual process of reconstruction, and this means that we need to trace how that reconstruction happens and we need to have a particular kind of methodological stance toward that. This is where we come to the deconstruction of pathology (see Parker, Georgaca, Harper, McLaughlin & Stowell Smith, 1995; Parker, 1999). What we accomplish in a deconstruction is simultaneously the production of something else. Let us return to Foucault for a moment. Reflecting on his studies of the dividing practices that constitute 'madness' as a certain kind of absence of 'reason', he says this, in an interview entitled 'Truth is in the Future':

> I am not merely an historian. I am not a novelist. What I do is a kind of historical fiction. In a sense I know very well that what I do is not true ... What I am trying to do is provoke an interference between our reality and the knowledge of our past history. If I succeed, this will have real effects in our present history. My hope is my books become true after they have been written—not before. (Foucault, 1980: 301) [22]

---

22. Thanks to Maria Nichterlein for drawing my attention to this reference.

We are now, then, diametrically opposed to an empiricist view of our objects of study, for we are now changing what it is we are examining, producing something new as we dismantle existing practices. A better way of putting it, though this admittedly is something that Foucault would not have been so happy with, is to say that we are 'dialectically opposed' to an empiricist view (Hook & Parker, 2002).

We need a different way of mapping 'mental health'. Maps of fantasy spaces can certainly be useful in freeing us from taken-for-granted assumptions about the world. However, the kind of map we need is one that will lead us from critical qualitative methodologies—the kind of semiological and genealogical studies that writers like Barthes and Foucault have been so useful for—toward a dialectical conception of research, which means that we do not merely interpret the world, but change it.

It is rather unfortunate that the Worker's Hall of Tampere is where Lenin met Stalin for the first time in 1905, and the approach I am advocating here is as much opposed to Stalinism as to contemporary neoliberal capitalist practice. However, as the website of the Tampere Lenin Museum, which is now the only permanent Lenin museum in the world, says, in a quote from Lenin, 'The decisive thing in Marxism is its revolutionary dialectic.'[23] Once again, the museum has a shop, for even Marxism can be commodified, and some very strange souvenirs are for sale, including some Lenin gloves which look as if they are designed for 'guerrilla gardening' (ecological activist interventions designed to question the built environment).

The revolutionary dialectic is a theoretical framework that is simultaneously directed at changing while interpreting. When we address questions of 'mental health' we are posed with the task of pairing deconstruction 'inside' psychology with deconstruction 'outside'. Dialectics here is not only a way of conceptualising what the deconstruction might be aiming at but it also helps us to understand the relation between the two domains and the two forms of critical work as not merely complementary but precisely as dialectical, as interwoven and contradictory, and as historically interlaced and as open to change.

We need to be able to distance ourselves from the temptation either to insert a truly dialectical psychology inside the disciplinary apparatuses that makes up the domain of mental health or to romanticise a real human psychology outside in psychological culture. The deconstruction of mental health is thus not a nihilistic enterprise but it is actually more 'constructive' than approaches that are merely tangled up in the day-to-day reconstruction of the boundaries between the normal and the pathological, so tangled up in those changing boundaries that they fail to help us think that there could be anything different beyond those taken-for-granted cultural horizons. The task of radical qualitative research into mental health should be to tackle those boundaries and help open the way to something better.

---

23. Tampere Lenin Museum, <http://www.lenin.fi/uusi/uk/index.htm> (accessed 7th June 2006).

REFERENCES

Barthes, R (1973) *Mythologies*. London: Paladin. (Original work published 1957)
Bilevsky, D (2006) 'Monster band has Finland fretting over face it shows.' *International Herald Tribune*, 22 May. Accessed 22 May 2006 at <http://www.iht.com/articles/2006/04/17/news/finn.php>
Blackman, L (1994) What is doing history? The use of history to understand the constitution of contemporary psychological objects. *Theory & Psychology, 4* (4), 485–504.
Booth, R & Smith, H (2006) 'Oh Lordi: From the land of Sibelius, a song for Satan.' *The Guardian*, 22 May, p 3.
Burman, E (2006) Emotions and reflexivity in feminised education action research. *Educational Action Research, 14* (3), 315–32.
Burman, E (2007) Between orientalism and normalisation: Cross-cultural lessons from Japan for a critical history of psychology. *History of Psychology, 16* (2), 179–98.
Crellin, C (1992) Whatever happened to plant psychology? *History and Philosophy of Psychology Newsletter, 15*, 25–32.
Evans, EP (1987) *The Criminal Prosecution and Capital Punishment of Animals: The lost history of Europe's animal trials*. London: Faber & Faber. (Original work published 1906)
Foucault, M (1980) Truth is in the future. In S Lotringer (Ed) *Foucault Live: Collected interviews, 1961–1984* (pp 298–301). New York: Semiotext(e).
Foucault, M (2006) *History of Madness*. London: Routledge.
Gordo López, AJ (2000) On the psychologization of critical psychology. *Annual Review of Critical Psychology, 2*, 55–71.
Harré, R (Ed) (1986) *The Social Construction of Emotion*. Oxford: Blackwell.
Hook, D & Parker, I (2002) Deconstruction, psychopathology and dialectics. *South African Journal of Psychology, 32* (2), 49–54.
Immelman, A (1999) Inside the mind of Milosevic, Unit for the Study of Personality in Politics. Accessed 16th June 2006 at <http://www.csbju.edu/uspp/Milosevic/Milosevic.html>.
Immelman, A (2003) Psychological profile of Saddam Hussein, Unit for the Study of Personality in Politics. Accessed 16th June 2006 at <http://www.csbju.edu/uspp/Research/Saddam%20profile.html>.
Parker, I (1995) Michel Foucault, psychologist. *The Psychologist, 8* (11), 503–5.
Parker, I (Ed) (1999) *Deconstructing Psychotherapy*. London: Sage.
Parker, I (2005) *Qualitative Psychology: Introducing radical research*. Buckingham: Open University Press.
Parker, I (2007) *Revolution in Psychology: Alienation to emancipation*. London: Pluto Press.
Parker, I (2008a) *Japan in Analysis: Cultures of the unconscious*. London: Palgrave.
Parker, I (2008b) Margins of resistance: Emotional illiteracy. *Qualitative Research in Psychology, 5*, 19–32.
Parker, I, Georgaca, E, Harper, D, McLaughlin, T & Stowell Smith, M (1995) *Deconstructing Psychopathology*. London: Sage.
Phoenix, A (1994) Practising feminist research: The intersection of gender and 'race' in the research process. In M Maynard & J Purvis (Eds) *Researching Women's Lives from a Feminist Perspective* (pp 49–71). London: Taylor & Francis.
Potter, J (1998) Fragments in the realization of relativism. In I Parker (Ed) *Social Constructionism, Discourse and Realism* (pp 27–45). London: Sage.

Robertson, R (1995) Glocalization: Time-space and homogeneity-heterogeneity. In M Featherstone, S Lash & R. Robertson (Eds) *Global Modernities* (pp 25–44). London: Sage Publications.

Sawacki, J (1991) *Disciplining Foucault: Feminism, power and the body.* London: Routledge.

Stanley, L & Wise, S (1983) *Breaking Out: Feminist consciousness and feminist research.* London: Routledge and Kegan Paul.

Ussher, J (1991) *Women's Madness: Misogyny or mental illness?* Hemel Hempstead: Harvester Wheatsheaf.

Wroe, S (2006) Letter in *The Guardian,* 23 May, p 33.

Yuval-Davis, N (2006) Intersectionality and feminist politics. *European Journal of Women's Studies, 13* (3), 193–209.

CHAPTER 4

THE AUTHORITY OF LIVED EXPERIENCE

ALASTAIR MORGAN

The concept of 'lived experience' has played a central role in discourses around mental health and mental distress. It has been particularly important in qualitative approaches to understanding the experiences of people suffering mental distress from their own perspective, and in providing a critical grounding for an attack on the dominant method of psychiatry as an abstraction from the lived experiences of service users. Diagnostic labelling, in particular, is viewed as a formal and abstract delineation of symptoms without any attention to the content of people's experiences. Psychiatry, as a discipline, is therefore erected upon a form/content division, which abstracts from the richness of individual experience to provide a formal description of modes of cognition and perception, where the content of thought is neither here nor there. This is most famously summed up in the statement by Kurt Schneider, the originator of the theory of front rank symptoms of psychosis, who stated that:

> Diagnosis looks for the 'How?' (form) not the 'What?' (the theme or content). When I find thought withdrawal, then this is important to me as a mode of inner experience and as a diagnostic hint, but it is not of diagnostic significance whether it is the devil, the girlfriend or a political leader who withdraws the thoughts. Wherever one focuses on such content diagnostics recedes: one sees then only the biographical aspects or existence open to interpretation. (cited in Bentall, 2004: 31)

Schneider's statement summarises a major strand of psychiatric theorising, one that sees form completely divided from content, and the delineation of form as the supreme task of any psychiatric hermeneutics. One thus dispenses with the superfluous and meaningless content as a mad rambling that is only of interest as an illumination of formal thought and affective disorder.

However, this is only one strand of theoretical psychiatry as it developed through the twentieth century, albeit a dominant one. The other two major elements of psychiatry— phenomenology and psychoanalysis—paid particular attention to content as meaningful, and as the proper subject of interpretation. Of course, one could argue that both Freud and Jaspers, as representatives of the psychoanalytic and phenomenological traditions within psychiatry, both banished madness proper, namely psychosis, from the realms of meaningfulness and understandability. This is undoubtedly so, but the manner of its exile only presaged a constant return in both traditions. Even within Jaspers' own argument around the 'ununderstandability' of psychotic states, there is a tension that calls into question the whole project of psychiatric hermeneutics. To adapt a phrase of Theodor Adorno, if one is to look for the 'experiential content' of both psychoanalysis and phenomenology as founding traditions of twentieth-century psychiatry, the struggle between reason and madness is inscribed deep within the practices of these traditions, even as they try to legislate their proper domains.[1] This is why the problem of madness returns with a vengeance. One only has to consider the main focus of so much phenomenological psychiatry after Jaspers, for example, the work of Minkowski and Binswanger, to take two salient examples, who both produced books on schizophrenia.

Nevertheless, despite this concern with experience, with content, it was only focused upon as an illumination of more profound and deep elements of the psyche. Content gives over to form in both the main traditions of psychoanalysis and phenomenology, in that a true understanding only arrives with the uncovering of fundamental structural elements of the life situation, whether these be unconscious desires, or deformations in the lived context of space and time. Lived experience itself, is only meaningful as the outward show of deeper forces. We could wonder whether we have moved any further from Schneider's account.

In recent years, there has been a renewed emphasis on the concept of a lived experience as the basis for understanding and working with mental distress. This has been framed without the deep structure/appearance or form/content divisions that dominated throughout twentieth-century psychiatry. Rather, the emphasis has been upon listening to the narratives of service users, on the sharing of common experiences, on understanding mental distress on a continuum model of mental experiences, and on normalising many experiences that had previously been termed pathological (see Anthony, 1993; Barker, 2001; Department of Health, 2001). Mental health services have been reoriented around models of recovery, that 'focus upon the "lived" or "real" life experience of the person' (Deegan: 2001: 15). Similarly, theorists have argued that there is a gulf between 'lived experiences and the accounts of mental health professionals' (Repper & Perkins, 2003: 4). The focus of ethical mental health work has shifted from the problem of interpretation and understanding, problems that were at the heart of twentieth-century psychiatry, to attempts to listen and absorb the meanings that people give to their own lives and their own narratives of their lives. Crucially, the concept of lived experience itself is not questioned or enquired into in any depth. The differentiation between surface meaning and deep structural significance is dispensed with in a form of postmodern pragmatism that prioritises only surface meaning, the meanings that people ascribe to their own lived experiences. A new discourse has arisen, with regards to lived

---

1. Adorno's concept of an experiential content to philosophy is outlined in many disparate sources, but can be clearly delineated in his essay entitled 'The Experiential content of Hegel's Philosophy', in Adorno, 1999.

experience, and it is a discourse that ascribes both an epistemic and moral authority to an unexamined concept of lived experience. What lived experiences are, we know very well, according to this discourse, because people tell us, and tell each other. It is this positivism of lived experience that I want to critically examine in this chapter. First, I want to outline what I consider to be the central epistemic and normative claims of this discourse on the authority of lived experience. Second, I want to examine the philosophical history of the concept of lived experience, in order to identify three very broad variants of the concept of lived experience. Third, I will relate these three variants to issues in mental health care, particularly to problems of interpretation and understanding, that I still feel should be central to the project of psychiatry. Finally, I want to return to the normative and epistemic claims of the authority of lived experience and to criticise them in a piecemeal fashion. I will do so in a piecemeal fashion, as I accept many of the claims of the authority of lived experience argument, but I think that there are certain issues that need to be considered in further depth.

THE EPISTEMIC AND NORMATIVE CLAIMS OF LIVED EXPERIENCE

The first and most important claim of the argument for the authority of lived experience is fundamentally epistemic; it relates to what is to count as knowledge when dealing in the sphere of mental health and mental distress. The claim is that lived experience is the evidential ground. It is the foundation and starting point of all our concerns and theorising in the field of mental health care. What this translates as, is that when researching in mental health or caring for the mentally distressed person, we must first be concerned with an accurate understanding of their own accounts of their experience, and it is these accounts that have evidential supremacy. In her famous article in the journal *Critical Inquiry*, Joan W. Scott (1991) examined this claim of the evidence of experience in relation to historical and literary studies, and in particular to histories of difference and of identity, when thinking of oppressed groups, be they women or lesbians and gay men, for example. Scott argues that narratives of experience in such accounts take on an evidential status that becomes the endpoint for any theorising. She writes:

> When the evidence offered is the evidence of 'experience', the claim for referentiality is further buttressed—what could be truer, after all, than a subject's own account of what he or she has lived through? (Scott, 1991: 777)

The claim for referentiality that Scott refers to is the problem that any account of reality is only a reflection or representation of reality which masks the process of its production as a representation. This problem is sidestepped in the argument that the accounts we give of our own experience are self-evidently true. This is the very claim that Scott contests in her article, arguing that such an appeal to the authority of experience, as an 'originary point of explanation', only masks fundamental questions about identity formation, and the society in which such an identity is formed. For Scott, such an argument for the authority of lived experience misses the Foucauldian point that:

> It is not individuals who have experience, but subjects who are constituted through experience. (Scott, 1991: 779)

However, such a definitive formulation itself masks a philosophical problem. To some degree, it makes sense to question what it means to have an experience, and to be formed as a subject within a process of constitution by powers and rules beyond our control. It is not enough to think that we can just dispense with the concept of experience and to talk instead of discourses and effects of power. There is still a question, as Foucault himself realised towards the end of his life, as to how we experience and appropriate our own selves as a crossing point for forces and powers and discourses of truth beyond our control.

In her recent book, Judith Butler has argued that what it means to give an account of ourselves, when we take into account the processes of constitutive structuring that take place in the formation of our identities, is to give an account of the losses and gaps at the heart of our selves. It is to give an account of those things that are not allowed into the particular regime of truth (Butler, 2005):

> [W]e are not simply the effects of discourses, but that any discourse, any regime of intelligibility, constitutes us at a cost. Our capacity to reflect upon ourselves, to tell the truth about ourselves is correspondingly limited by what the discourse, the regime, cannot allow into speakability. (Butler, 2005: 121)

What cannot be allowed to be spoken is literally unspeakable, and so Butler moves to psychoanalysis as a practice par excellence that can allow an absence to come to light. Of course, all of this talk of absences coming to light is as far away from the positivism of the authority of lived experience argument as you can get. What I want to state here is that one cannot claim narratives of self-experience as some kind of fact or evidential ground without an interpretation and examination of the forces that constitute and allow them into speakability. This does not mean, I think, that we are just effects of discourse and that we can dispense completely with the concept of experience, but it does mean that we have to take into account the gaps and fissures at the heart of our experiences and our accounts of our experiences. It also means that the idea that our lived experiences are somehow individually owned, transparent and easy to give an account of, an idea that lies at the heart of the argument about the authority of lived experience, cannot be held to uncritically.

I have spent some time on this central claim for the evidence of experience because I think it lies at the core of the argument for a certain authority of lived experience, and it also tends towards a positivism about lived experiences, as though they were something one could grasp and relate to in a quite straightforward manner. However, there are further epistemic claims that flow from this central argument for lived experience as evidential ground. First is the argument that our research and practice in the mental health field should get closer to starting from and prioritising the experiences of service users. I agree with this as an epistemic claim, although I will argue that it is complicated by my earlier critique of the idea of lived experience as evidential ground. Second is the argument that the means to getting closer to experience, the prescribed methodology, is one of collecting narratives, encouraging self-help groups, and creating spaces for users/carers to share views. Again, I think this is vitally important, but should also be questioned as the *ne plus ultra* of mental health research and practice. Finally, there is the strong epistemic claim that people who have shared experiences can better understand each other. This claim can come in either weak or strong varieties. The weak variety does not claim an exclusivity to understanding based upon shared experience, whereas the strong version does. Therefore, the strong version of the argument will run that only people who have shared experiences can truly understand one another. At some level, this is, of course, true. A commonality of experience, particularly a commonality of the experience of being a recipient of mental health services, and of the discrimination and stigma that go along with labels of mental illness, provides a powerful basis for fighting discrimination and oppression. However, this argument should not completely obscure the reality that experiences are not as similar and straightforward that simply sharing will provide appropriate understanding and support. Furthermore, this argument tends to obscure the central problem of interpretation within psychiatry. The problem of reason understanding madness, even understanding its own madness, is occluded in a discourse of shared identities and common experiences. The cost of this, I think, is that an unthinking pragmatism domesticates experiences that are, in some sense, radically ununderstandable, but still demand understanding. I will return to this argument later. Following from these central epistemic claims about the authority of lived experience, there are a number of normative claims that serve as a critique of psychiatry and as injunctions for a different form of mental health care.

There are three central normative claims. First, is the argument that in mental health care, the lived experiences of service users have been fundamentally disregarded and ignored. Similarly, the project of understanding in psychiatry has proceeded through the suppression of individual lived experiences. Finally, mental health care should be reoriented so that it takes into account service users' views, and voices at the centre of their own care. I agree with these three normative claims. Therefore, my critique is targeted at certain epistemological questions about the nature of lived experiences. However, I do think that these epistemological questions will impact upon how we might reconsider these normative claims, a reconsideration that I will return to at the end of the chapter.

In this opening section, then, I have outlined what I consider to be the central epistemic and normative claims for the argument for the authority of lived experience, and I have specifically questioned the central claim of the evidence of lived experience, which I argue leads to a certain positivism about what lived experience is. In the next section, I want to consider in more detail what the concept of 'lived experience' really means, and I will do this through a conceptual history of the terms, which will demonstrate that it means many things to many people.

THE CONCEPT OF LIVED EXPERIENCE

The concept of a lived experience sounds intuitively odd to English ears. Even more so, the affirmations involved in phrases such as a 'real, lived experience', or an 'actual, lived experience'. The temptation is to respond by querying what an experience could or would be that was not lived in some sense, and then why we need this peculiar designation of a 'lived experience'.

The straightforward answer to such questions lies in the problem of translation from German philosophical vocabulary. There are two words for experience used within German philosophy, *Erfahrung* and *Erlebnis*.

The concept of experience as *Erfahrung*, which is historically prior to the appearance of the word *Erlebnis* at the end of the nineteenth century, has two distinct usages in German philosophy. First, there is the epistemological usage that reaches its apotheosis in Kant's philosophy. *Erfahrung* is the description of the cognitive experience involved in judgement and knowledge. The process in the Kantian concept of experience, whereby a unified subject orders and classifies the raw data of experience, is a process that can be termed experience as a whole. This experience, then, is the process whereby an inert objectivity is synthesised by a subject and raw sensations are formed into the object of experience. In some sense, experience is configured here as a junior partner to the understanding, in that, in the Kantian sense that there is no knowledge without experience, but experience without the synthesising operations of subjective judgement could not be termed experience at all. Kant's attempt to chart a path between rationalism and empiricism results in a concept of experience which is concerned with the limits and possibilities of reason itself. These limits and possibilities are modelled upon the dominant modes of scientific reasoning of the time (the certitude of mathematical and geometrical reasoning). Experience relates to the knowledge we have of the world but is bounded within the possibilities available to our faculty of understanding. Therefore, we cannot know things as they are in themselves, but only as they appear and are synthesised within the categories of the human understanding. Experience, here, attempts two distinct and important philosophical tasks; the modelling of a human reasoning upon the certitude of the natural sciences, and a drawing of the boundaries for the possibility of experience, within the realm of empirical knowledge. For Kant, experience lies in a conjunction of conceptual understanding and empirical intuition, which results in an orderly pattern of knowledge and reason.[2]

The second way that *Erfahrung* develops as a concept of experience is in contrast with the Kantian idea of experience and more indebted to Hegel's philosophy, particularly his work, *Phenomenology of Spirit* (1977). This is the more historically inflected idea of experience, an idea of experience as a journey, a learning process, that is individual, but dependent upon a tradition and a community. An experience, in this sense, is an achievement, an accomplishment that only arrives through an immersion in a culture

---

2. The importance of Kant as a philosopher is that his thought constantly pushes against its own limits. So, although he attempted to limit reason within the bounds of a possible (continued overleaf)

and tradition, which allows for a departure through the accumulated and assimilated experience of such a tradition. Such a concept of experience presumes an individual who is able over time to order and unify an experience through an accumulated memory and sedimentation of tradition and community.[3] Experience, in this sense, develops its own limits and possibilities through its historical progress and through its appearance in histories. Thus, for Hegel, experience becomes a progression through various forms of historical consciousness, which arrives at an absolute truth that is immanent within each stage, but not yet fully developed. Hegel overturns the Kantian limits of experience, with an account of how experience can develop and overcome its limits through a historical progression of reason.

It was in response to these two concepts of experience that the concept of *Erlebnis* arose in German philosophy in the late nineteenth century (see Jay, 2005: 95–96, 222). Gadamer (1989) outlines the history of the term *Erlebnis* in his book, *Truth and Method*. He writes that as a noun the term first came to prominence in the 1870s, when it was used in biographical writing. *Erlebnis*, with its use of the prefix 'er-', added to the word for 'living', *lebnis*, gives a deepening sense to the verb that follows it, carrying the sense of a deepening of life, as Gadamer says the 'immediacy with which something is grasped' (Gadamer, 1989: 61). There is a clear link between the terminology of *Erlebnis*, which first enters concrete philosophical usage with Dilthey, and the life philosophy developed by Nietzsche and Bergson, which served as a philosophical critique of scientific, positivist thought by privileging modes of experiencing which are in some sense deeper than the rational formulations of enlightenment thought. Dilthey attempted to articulate a form of experience that would literally revivify philosophy. He characterises previous philosophy of experience in the following manner:

> There is no real blood flowing in the veins of the knowing subject fabricated by Locke, Hume and Kant, but rather the diluted lymph of reason as mere intellectual activity. (Dilthey, 1988: 173)

The concept of *Erlebnis* arose in a reaction against the restriction of reason to a narrow, cognitive and instrumental form of experience. The Kantian attempt to model experience upon a grounding in the forms of certainty characteristic of the natural sciences was seen as a radical reduction and dehumanisation of experience. This reaction coalesced in the latter part of the nineteenth century into a loose grouping of philosophers concerned with life philosophy, or *Lebensphilosophie*. Life philosophy has been associated with a

---

(continued) experience in the first critique, the second and third critiques, which deal with morality and aesthetic judgement, demonstrate the limits of this approach. For an excellent discussion of Kant's philosophy in the light of this tension, see Adorno's posthumously published lectures (Adorno, 2001) on Kant, particularly *Kant's Kritik der Reinen Vernunft, Nachgelassene Schriften, 4,* Frankfurt am Main: Suhrkamp Verlag (see Kant, 1989).

3. There are numerous discussions of *Erfahrung*, some of which are cited in the text as the concept is analysed in more detail. One of the best discussions of both *Erfahrung* and *Erlebnis* is contained in Gadamer, 1989.

group of philosophers from the end of the nineteenth century, particularly Nietzsche, Dilthey and Bergson (Palmer, 1969).[4] However, the broad concerns of life philosophy were passed down from the Romanticism of the eighteenth century, from thinkers such as Herder, Novalis, Schiller and Schelling. Philosophies of life broadly shared a concern with a delineation of (often configured as a return to) the full experiential richness of life in opposition to technological, schematised modes of human thought. This occasionally accompanied forms of vitalism that verged on mystic irrational thought about the foundational psychic energy of life, but also emphasised a concrete thinking in terms of starting from human experience itself. There was a fundamental division in terms of whether the life that was being considered was human life or life in itself. For example, Bergson, and in a different way Nietzsche, were particularly concerned with life, and the forces of life itself, in how they structured human existence and produced new forms of existence regardless of human agency. Dilthey was more concerned with the interpretation of human forms of experience through the construction of a philosophy of interpretation, which did not suppress the living material at hand but philosophised from experience itself. What these writers shared was a critique of experience in modernity and a concern with a thinking about life as something that has been suppressed by modern forms of thought and modes of understanding.

The concept of *Erlebnis* achieved its most rigorous formulation in the philosophical movement of phenomenology. It was in the work of Edmund Husserl spanning the first thirty years of the twentieth century that phenomenology developed a philosophy of lived experience that attempted to systematically distinguish itself from either rationalism or empiricism.[5] Phenomenology attempted to investigate the nature of experience through a delineation of the ways in which phenomena appear to consciousness. Rather than concerning itself with the problem of how the mind reaches out to the world, or how sensations get into the mind, phenomenology concerned itself with a consciousness that was always already in the world, consciousness as fundamentally intentional, a consciousness of something. This form of experience always lies beyond any subject–object differentiation, and cannot be encompassed through the model of the certitude of the natural sciences. Furthermore, for Husserl, the natural attitude we take towards our world already masks this structure of consciousness as a consciousness of something, as intentionality. Husserl attempted, what he termed the transcendental *epoché*, the bracketing out of all our normal taken-for-granted perceptions of the world, to try and achieve an originary lived experience of the world.

For Husserl this bracketing of everyday experience tends to get configured in rationalist terms, in the terms of a transcendental consciousness which can be uncovered as the unity of intending consciousness with intended object. However, later phenomenology, particularly the early work of Martin Heidegger and the work of Merleau-Ponty, viewed this originary, primordial lived experience in terms of bodily situation, practical activity and a fundamental subjectivity or owning of experience. For

---
4. For an excellent brief discussion of *Lebensphilosophie*, see Schnädelbach, 1984.
5. To complicate matters, it would have to be admitted that Husserl moved between using the term *Erfahrung* and the term *Erlebnis*.

Merleau-Ponty, experience is always embodied and situated before it is knowledge. This embodiment is always implied in any way of knowing the world. But, this fundamental situatedness of experience, this lived experience, cannot be easily grasped or thematised using the conceptual tools of language. Our knowledge and experience rests on a basis of lived experience that cannot be reduced to the forms of rationality that we impose, but nor can it be immediately experienced or appropriated. In a discussion, Merleau-Ponty articulates this point well:

> Assuredly a life is not a philosophy. I thought I had indicated in passing that description is not the return to immediate experience; one never returns to immediate experience. It is only a question of whether we are to try to understand it. I believe that to attempt to express immediate experience is not to betray reason, but, on the contrary to work toward its aggrandizement … It is to begin the effort of expression and of what is expressed: it is to accept the condition of a beginning reflection. (Merleau-Ponty, 1964: 12–27)

Merleau-Ponty uses the idea of a lived experience in terms of our embodied situation, as the basis for all other forms of experience, but, it is a basis that can only be expressed in philosophy and never completely grasped in its immediacy.

To sum up certain key aspects of this first broad concept of lived experience, before moving on. Lived experience refers to an unreflective, immediately transparent, individual experience. It encompasses emotion, feeling, suffering, desire and volition. In Husserl's phenomenology this originary form of pre-reflective lived experience is theorised initially as a form of essential evidencing intuition which grounds all thought. However, in Husserl's later work, and in the appropriation of phenomenology by Heidegger and Merleau-Ponty, this pre-reflective lived experience is conceived as a fundamental way of being-in-the-world, the way that the world is given to us as embodied engaged beings.

However, although this lived experience is a primary pre-reflective experience, it can only be reflected upon through the means of conceptual representation. This is why Merleau-Ponty stresses the point that phenomenology is always 'the beginning of a continuing reflection'. We cannot grasp the immediacy of our core lived experiences, but only reflect upon them in a second-hand manner. Thus, there is a tension within the concept of lived experience, as something that is primary and fundamental, but also impossible to formulate in a representational or conceptual manner. The question is how we can move from this individual, affective, pre-reflective core of experience to its formulation in either an individual narrative unity or in terms of a shared culture, without sacrificing the supposed immediacy and particularity of lived experience to the realm of law, in the way that Kant's philosophy is purported to do.

One means of responding to this tension has taken place within a strand of thought about lived experience that embraces the problem of representation. This could be termed the second concept of lived experience. In this concept of lived experience, experience is embraced as something that breaks the bounds of any form of conceptual representation. It is viewed in terms of limit experiences, which break the bounds of the everyday.

This concept of lived experience can be viewed even within phenomenology itself. If the originary unity of subject and object cannot be grasped through conceptual reasoning, then philosophy calls for a form of heightened consciousness removed from the everyday. The transcendental *epoché* that Husserl describes already prefigures this search for an experience that moves beyond the bounds of possible experience. The second form of *Erlebnis* is that experience that, either as revealed in terms of religious experience, or in terms of aesthetic or surrealist experience, would move beyond everyday forms of temporality and continuities of chronological time and personal identity over time. There is a sense of this experience in Heidegger's account of an authentic appropriation of certain fundamental moods which open up the possibility of the experience of different forms of temporality as a projection into the future (Heidegger, 1993). One could also think of the Bergsonian concept of *durée* as an access to a different and deeper relation of lived experience. This form of lived experience then gives access to a deeper truth about life itself, removed from the instrumental modes of thinking characteristic of everyday rationalities. It is through an experience that tests the limits of experience itself that a lived experience can find its truth.

This idea of an experience beyond the everyday, of heightened and intensified experiences, plays a central role in much French philosophy of the mid to late twentieth century. Experience here is fundamentally discontinuous, ununderstandable, and yet, liberating.[6] A range of philosophers and artists theorise a series of experiences such as erotic experiences, suffering, pain, war, religious/spiritual experiences, madness, dying (or more specifically, the moment of death). These experiences are viewed as fundamentally unnarratable or, in some sense, breaking the bonds of representation. They also dispense with the idea of a subject owning experience. Whereas the first concept of experience thinks of lived experience as essentially constitutive of subjectivity at its very core, these experiences somehow dislocate and dislodge the very idea of a subjective ownership of experience.

Finally, with this second concept of lived experience, the idea of a lived experience as a form of excess or escape is aligned with a concept of freedom. This idea of a limit experience is viewed as a route beyond the constraints of subject formation and conceptual representation, to the revelation of deeper truths about experience itself.

As a reaction to this discourse of *Erlebnis* in early twentieth-century German philosophy, a group of Marxist-inspired philosophers, known retrospectively as the Frankfurt School, developed a quite distinctive usage of the concept of lived experience. They were very sceptical of the notion of any immediate experience itself, and acutely aware of the dangers of a fetishisation of heightened, intense experiences for their own sake, as they saw in the political climate of the 1930s in Germany how these experiences could be manipulated to a catastrophic effect. It was Walter Benjamin, who was loosely affiliated to the Frankfurt School, who most eloquently developed a concept of *Erlebnis* which had a far more critical and pessimistic hue than that bestowed upon it by life

---

6. One thinks of Bataille, particularly in this regard (see Bataille, 1988), but it is also a central theme in both Foucault and Deleuze's philosophy. For an interesting discussion, see Jay (1995).

philosophy and phenomenology. In his work on Baudelaire, Benjamin thematises the transition in modern experience through a differentiation between *Erlebnis* and *Erfahrung* (Benjamin, 1997). The problem, for Benjamin, in this relationship between *Erfahrung* and *Erlebnis* is the place of tradition in modernity. It is the distinctive mode of experience within modernity that it has lost its relation to tradition. Benjamin argues that the increasing technological sophistication of society has produced forms of communication which have atrophied the possibility of experience, in the sense of *Erfahrung* (Benjamin, 1999). The replacement of narration by information has atrophied the possibility of authority in the tradition of communicable experience. Alongside this are the increasing shocks, both on an everyday basis and on a larger basis in modern society, which do not enable the individual to assimilate experiences. In 'The Storyteller', Benjamin refers to soldiers returning from the First World War, without the possibility of communicating their experience (Benjamin, 1999: 84). In the essay on Baudelaire, he refers to the everyday shocks of modern city living which preclude the individual from assimilating experience. Using Freud's essay 'Beyond the Pleasure Principle', Benjamin cites the necessity for the human organism to be constantly alert to the parrying of shocks to its perceptual system. The greater the shocks are in the perceptual system, the more human consciousness becomes an alert system which parries the shocks that are surrounding it, and the less do these impressions enter into the perceptual apparatus and become lasting experiences:

> The greater the share of the shock factor in particular impressions the more constantly consciousness has to be alert as a screen against stimuli: the more efficiently it is so, the less do these impressions enter experience (Erfahrung) tending to remain in the sphere of a certain hour in one's life (Erlebnis).
> (Benjamin, 1997: 117)

What Benjamin argues in the essay on Baudelaire and in the 'Storyteller' essay is that with the onset of modernity and, particularly, with the First World War, there was what John McCole terms an 'epochal upheaval in the human sensorium' (McCole, 1993: 1). It is this change in experience that Benjamin equates with *Erlebnis*, in the sense that with the constant shocks of city life, the human perceptual organism is unable to assimilate sensations and form a stock of experience. There is a correspondence between the shock experience of everyday city life, the worker's experience at the machine and the bombardment of information that replaces the processes of narration. All of these shocks combine to atrophy modern experience.

What Benjamin recognised in the period between the two wars was a change in the structure of experience itself, that lived experience cannot be presented as a ground for experience without a realisation of shifts and transformations in the structure of that experience, shifts which can, as Benjamin described, be dramatic and traumatic. In a stronger sense, Critical Theory viewed lived experience as a decayed or damaged form of experience. Writers such as Benjamin, Theodor Adorno, and Herbert Marcuse were interested in articulating the ways in which our very core and basic experiences of the world around us had been infiltrated by the capitalist forms of production and reproduction of social life. Particularly, in an analysis of the commodity form and how it structures even our core, affective life, these thinkers developed a distinctive concept of lived experience as fundamentally reified.

Drawing on Georg Lukács's concept of reification developed in his seminal text, *History and Class Consciousness*, written in 1919, the Frankfurt School argue that human lived experiences, rather than being the fluid, unrepresentable instances of freedom, have rather been turned into analogies of commodities, infinitely exchangeable artifacts (Lukács, 1971). In his book, *Minima Moralia*, which is subtitled 'Reflections from Damaged Life', Theodor Adorno constructs an immanent critique of everyday life through an enumeration of examples of lived experiences which have all become marked and deformed by the processes of exchange and abstraction marked by capitalist society. Our modes of dealing with objects, greeting people, exchanging presents, forming attachments are all viewed with a mordant eye, as instances of total commodification. Rather than the apotheosis of freedom, lived experience here becomes the site for a hermeneutic of damage and decay (Adorno, 1997).[7]

Therefore, for these thinkers from the Frankfurt School, lived experience takes on an eminently differing hue from the two earlier concepts of lived experience that were outlined above. Rather, than a constitutive core of experience, or a libidinal excess of experience, lived experience is theorised as a decayed husk, even in its affective responses to intersubjectivity and objectivity. Furthermore, lived experience is certainly not transparent and immediate. Many of the analyses of lived experience undertaken by Frankfurt School thinkers are focused upon an unmasking of supposedly ahistorical forms of pre-reflective existence as fundamentally historically structured through capitalist forms of production and reproduction of social life. It is only through a critical view taken upon lived experience that the possibility of an unmasking of the forces at work that structure our experience can be undertaken. Lived experience is also not viewed as individual, but as an index of a damaged whole. Individual experience can only be viewed through the social form in which it arises.

Furthermore, there can be no escape from such a reified existence. Adorno, in particular, argued that even our free time and practices of cultural consumption, are, in themselves infiltrated by structures of commodity exchange. There is no simple route beyond such a reified society, and the invocation of libidinal excess, so beloved of the advocates of the second concept of lived experience, does not take into account how our very affects and desires are structured within a consumer society. Lived experience is therefore, the starting point for the particular hermeneutic procedure of the Frankfurt School, rather than its fundamental basis. Any talk about authentic or true lived experience is itself an ideological stance which masks fundamental injustices in society.

---

7. For an extended discussion of the concept of damaged life in relation to Adorno's work, see my discussion in Morgan (2007).

THREE FORMS OF LIVED EXPERIENCE

From this very brief conceptual history, I have rather crudely developed three strands of the concept of lived experience. I will admit that this philosophical history tends to gloss over many problems and complexities, but my purpose here is to bring these three strands of the concept of lived experience to bear on the argument for the authority of lived experience when thinking about and working in mental health care.

The first concept of lived experience refers to an immediate, pre-reflective, affective experience of everyday life. There is a constant tension in this concept of lived experience between its immediacy and the narrative accumulation of such experiences into 'a life', or 'a society'. However, these experiences are individually owned, transparent, and incontestable in the sense that they are self-evidently true. I take this to be the concept of lived experience that predominantly lies behind the authority of the lived experience argument that we examined earlier. However, I don't think that the tension between immediacy and narrative is really acknowledged to any great degree when this concept is appropriated.

The second concept of lived experience refers to transcendent, often libidinal, experiences that burst the bonds of the everyday. These experiences cannot be owned, or even represented or narrated in a conventional sense.

The third and final concept of lived experience refers to the damaged and degraded experience of everyday life that means that our core, affective responses to the world are infiltrated at a very basic level by the dictates of modern, capitalist society. Similarly to the second concept, these experiences cannot be theorised as individually owned in any sense, but in contrast with the second concept they are supremely immanent rather than transcendent and indicative of damage rather than freedom.

What, then, is the relevance of this conceptual history and the excavation of these three strands of the concept of lived experience to theory and practice in mental health care? First, I think when writing about lived experience and mental health, we should take account of the multiple meanings of the concept of lived experience, and, at least try and situate our usage of this concept within this philosophical history. In relation to the first form of lived experience, I think it is right to argue that an individual's account of what has happened to them is epistemically privileged in a certain manner. It does seem both morally and intuitively wrong for our first reaction to a person's account of their own experience to be one of contestation and denial.

However, we should be aware of how the process of giving such an account will involve both conscious and unconscious omissions; that there is always a gap between experience and the reconstruction of experience. Therefore, I would contest the argument that lived experience is transparent and self-evident.

Finally, I would argue that lived experience is neither straightforwardly owned nor narratable. The metaphor of ownership of experience, or an expertise from experience, treats experience as though it were some form of identifiable property that can be easily identified and assimilated. Similarly, any narration of experience has to take into account the problems of representation involved, and the form in which the account takes place.

In relation to the second concept of experience, a whole ream of questions are opened up when we reflect upon its relevance for the subject of mental health and mental distress. First, is the question of whether the experience of madness can ever be narrated. Second, is the question of the relationship between madness and the self, particularly when thinking about the concept of recovery. When we are talking about recovery from schizophrenia, are we thinking about a unitary personal identity over time, that recovers a true self after a dispossession of self during a psychotic phase, or does a new self arise in an integrative sense after the absorption of some meaning in psychosis? To answer such questions would obviously take more space than is available here, but my purpose is to raise the complexity of using a concept of lived experience when referring, say, to recovery from psychosis, when the very experience of psychosis itself will pose the question of the subject of such a lived experience. Finally, there are problems of capacity and coercion that are constantly raised within mental health care. If mental health care is always to begin from an understanding of the lived experience of the service user, then how do we justify care provision which then imposes something upon a person against their will, but in their best interests? Are we arguing that their true self lies behind the experience of mental distress, and therefore they lack capacity and can be coerced? If we are doing this, then the argument for authority of lived experience becomes very much more complicated than it appears at first. At certain times, we start from the lived experiences of service users but at others we have a sense of what are false experiences and what are not. However, if we decide to always take each lived experience at face value, then there can be no problem of capacity at all, and therefore no mitigation if someone with a mental disorder commits a crime. These traditional problems of mental health care do not disappear with the argument for the authority of lived experience.

If we take into account the third form of lived experience, then the very transparency and immediacy of lived experience is brought into question. Experiences, including experiences of mental distress, need to be related to their appearance within a particular form of society and culture. Furthermore, lived experience should not always be conceptualised in individual terms, but related to the structures which enable and suppress the formation of identities. In the introduction to the collection of essays he edited entitled *Critical Psychiatry*, David Ingleby outlines two hermeneutic procedures with regards to the project of understanding within psychiatry. The first, which he terms 'normalizing', gives an account of what is happening in the terms of what the person feels or thinks is happening. It privileges the accounts of the service user themselves. The second interpretive approach, that he terms, along with Habermas, a 'depth hermeneutics', are interpretations which 'actively criticise and transcend people's own understanding of themselves' (Ingleby, 1981: 47). Any interpretation that takes seriously this third form of lived experience will clearly operate at some level of depth hermeneutics, of an attempt to transcend and actively criticize self-understandings. This raises the difficult question of a paternalism in critical interpretation itself, that has led to concepts such as false consciousness, or ideology critique becoming outmoded in critical discourse because they are felt to be paternalistic. However, the alternative of a simple acceptance of a positivistically uncritical concept of lived experience itself carries the dangers of just entrenching an individualised notion of experience that has its own ideological problems.

THE AUTHORITY OF LIVED EXPERIENCE

Where does this all leave the argument for the authority of lived experience that we began with? Well, I think it leaves intact the idea that we must begin with the accounts people give of their experience. Any theory or practice in mental health that fundamentally bypasses or abstracts from the experiences that people give an account of is in some way going to produce an interpretation that is damaging or fundamentally wrong.

Furthermore, we can accept, that, at some level, people with shared experiences will have a fundamentally more empathic and therefore deeper understanding of the issues that they face.

However, I don't think that these arguments are the final word in terms of mental health care and theory, and I don't feel that they fundamentally solve some of the central antinomies of psychiatry. In fact, their use as an ideology of lived experience tends to mask the fundamental tensions that continue unabated in day-to-day mental health care.

The problems of interpretation and understanding remain within mental health care. It is never sufficient to just listen and absorb a narrative of experience without attempting to understand that experience in relation to a personal identity over time (alongside discontinuities within that identity), and the relationship between that identity and the society within which it has been formed. Furthermore, we have to accept, taking our cue from the second form of lived experience, that not all experiences, particularly limit experiences such as madness, can be amenable to simple narration and representation.

Therefore, lived experiences can and, at times, should be contested. Of course, this opens up the question of who has the right to contest and when can they contest. On what authority can someone contest someone else's experience. Surely, many of the abuses of psychiatry have rested upon the arrogation of authority by a medical establishment that, on dubious grounds, has decided that it can decide between norm and pathology. This is true, but I think it is a tension that cannot be wished away. Psychiatry, at some level, will always be a 'monologue of reason about madness', to use Foucault's oft-quoted formulation, but the ethics of psychiatry lie within an understanding and acceptance of the difficulties inherent to the task of the attempt to understand, and always failing to understand, madness as a social and historical form of life (see Foucault, 1993: xii–xiii).

The normative claims of the argument for lived experience still hold as a critique of the abstracting and dominating practices of psychiatry, but the treatment of lived experience as a foundationalist given, and the account of experience as a journey of recovery are metaphors that only serve to entrench a superficial, individualist ethos that, in itself, occludes any critical investigation of the relationships between mental distress and society.

REFERENCES

Adorno, TW (1997) *Minima Moralia. Reflections from damaged life* (EFN Jephcott, Trans). London/New York: Verso.

Adorno, TW (1999) *Hegel: Three studies* (S Weber Nicholsen, Trans). Cambridge, MA/London: MIT Press.

Adorno, TW (2001) *Kant's Critique of Pure Reason,* R Tiedemann (Ed) (R Livingstone, Trans). Cambridge: Polity Press.

Anthony, WA (1993) Recovery from mental illness: The guiding vision of the mental health service in the 1990s. *Psychosocial Rehabilitation Journal, 16,* 11–23.

Barker, P (2001) The Tidal Model: Developing an empowering, person-centred approach to recovery within psychiatric and mental health nursing. *Journal of Psychiatric and Mental Health Nursing, 8* (3), 233–40.

Bataille, G (1988) *Inner Experience* (LA Boldt, Trans). Albany, NY: SUNY Press.

Benjamin, W (1997) *Charles Baudelaire: A lyric poet in the era of high capitalism* (H Zohn, Trans). London/New York: Verso.

Benjamin, W (1999) The storyteller. In *Illuminations* (H Zohn, Trans). London: Pimlico.

Bentall, R (2003) *Madness Explained: Psychosis and human nature.* London: Penguin.

Bergson, H (2002), *Key Writings,* K Ansell-Pearson & J Mullarkey (Eds). New York/London: Continuum.

Butler, J (2005) *Giving an Account of Oneself.* New York: Fordham University Press.

Deegan, P (2001) Recovery as a self-directed process of healing and transformation. *Occupational Therapy in Mental Health, 17* (3&4), 15–21.

Deleuze, G & Guattari, F (1988) *A Thousand Plateaus: Capitalism and schizophrenia* (B Massumi, Trans). London: The Athlone Press.

Department of Health (2001) *The Journey to Recovery: The government's vision for mental health care.* London: DoH.

Dilthey, W (1988) *Introduction to the Human Sciences: An attempt to lay a foundation for the study of society and history* (RJ Betanzos, Trans). Detroit, MI: Wayne State University Press.

Foucault, M (1993) *Madness and Civilisation.* London: Routledge.

Foucault, M (1998) A preface to transgression. In JD Faubion (Ed) *Aesthetics, Method and Epistemology: The essential works, 1954–1984* (R Hurley et al., Trans). London: Allen Lane, Penguin Press.

Gadamer, H-G (1989) *Truth and Method* (J Weinsheimer & DG Marshall, Trans). London: Sheed and Ward.

Hegel, GWF (1977) *Phenomenology of Spirit* (AV Miller, Trans) with a foreword by JN Findlay. Oxford/New York/Melbourne: Oxford University Press.

Heidegger, M (1993) *Being and Time* (J Macquarrie and E Robinson, Trans). Oxford/Cambridge, MA: Blackwell.

Husserl, E (1960) *Cartesian Meditations* (D Cairns, Trans). The Hague: Nijhoff.

Husserl, E (1970) *The Crisis of the European Sciences and Transcendental Phenomenology: An introduction to phenomenological philosophy* (D Carr, Trans). Evanston, IL: Northwestern University Press.

Ingleby, D (1981) Understanding 'mental illness'. In D Ingleby (Ed) *Critical Psychiatry: The politics of mental health* (pp 23–71). Harmondsworth: Penguin.

Jay, M (1995) The limits of limit experience. *Constellations, 2* (2), 159–67.

Jay, M (2005) *Songs of Experience. Modern American and European variations on a universal theme.* Berkeley, CA/London: University of California Press.

Kant, I (1989) *Critique of Pure Reason* (N Kemp Smith, Trans). London: Macmillan.

Lukács, G (1971) *History and Class Consciousness: Studies in Marxist dialectics* (R Livingstone, Trans). London: Merlin Press.

McCole, J (1993) *Walter Benjamin and the Antinomies of Tradition.* Ithaca, NY/London: Cornell University Press.

Merleau-Ponty, M (1964) *The Primacy of Perception and Other Essays* (JM Edie, Trans). Evanston, IL: Northwestern University Press.

Merleau-Ponty, M (1989) *Phenomenology of Perception* (C Smith, Trans). London: Routledge.

Morgan, A (2007) *Adorno's Concept of Life.* London/New York: Continuum.

Palmer, RE (1969) *Hermeneutics: Interpretation and theory in Schleiermacher, Dilthey, Heidegger and Gadamer.* Evanston, IL: Northwestern University Press.

Repper, J & Perkins, R (2003) *Social Inclusion and Recovery: A model for mental health practice.* London: Ballière Tindall.

Rickman, HP (1979) *Wilhelm Dilthey: Pioneer of the human sciences.* London: Paul Elek.

Schnädelbach, H (1984) *Philosophy in Germany: 1831–1933* (E Matthews, Trans). Cambridge/London/New York: Cambridge University Press.

Scott, JW (1991) The evidence of experience. *Critical Inquiry, 17,* 773–97.

Chapter 5

PHILOSOPHY AND PSYCHE
WHAT CAN PHILOSOPHY TELL PSYCHIATRY, PSYCHOLOGY AND PSYCHOTHERAPY?

Miles Clapham

INTRODUCTION

'Philosophy changes nothing and leaves everything as it is.' Wittgenstein's (1993a) statement might seem to confirm many people's prejudice that philosophy has little to offer, especially in an intensely practical field such as medicine. One thing the statement may be taken to imply is an ethical position of profound respect for whatever it is being examined. Wittgenstein here as elsewhere is setting out the limits of the field, although he may be taken as disingenuous, as his intent seems to be to change the way we think, or at least examine it critically. Wittgenstein saw philosophy as a therapy that could undo the false pictures we have of the world and of ourselves, and so reduce confusion and the suffering this can induce. In some ways his method has a kinship with cognitive behavioural therapy (CBT) in its challenging of misleading or distressing ways of thinking, but Wittgenstein's enquiry goes further.

Wittgenstein did not found a school of therapy, although he did offer a method of dealing with these false ideas. He showed that a careful interrogation of language and how we speak undoes false or mistaken ways of thinking. He particularly wanted to show that the 'ordinary' use of language was full of wisdom, and the 'technical' use of language in philosophy leads to confusion, because it seeks to pin things down in ways that end up mystifying people (Heaton, 2000a; Stroll, 2002). Wittgenstein was interested in Freud, and thought that Freud's theories were a prime example of the misuse of language, with dangerous consequences (Heaton, 2000a).

In this chapter I will introduce three related areas that appear in Wittgenstein's and some other twentieth-century philosophers' thinking that have the most direct relevance to psychiatry, psychology and psychotherapy. First, is the limit of scientific or theoretical understandings of the mind, and how ordinary language allows us to understand ourselves and other people. Then I will look at the nature and central importance of ethics to these fields, particularly in psychotherapy where the ethical aspects of the relationship are perhaps most important for how the therapy goes. Finally I will say something about the possibilities and limits of therapeutic language.

As well as Wittgenstein, Heidegger has much to contribute when considering language and the nature of thinking. Kierkegaard is important both because of his influence on later philosophers, and because of his profound descriptions of various styles of existence such as anxiety and despair.

THE LIMITS OF SCIENTIFIC UNDERSTANDING OF 'THE MIND'

Wittgenstein's initial work, first published in 1921, the *Tractatus Logico-Philosophicus* (1961), was concerned with both the sorts of things science can say through logical propositions, and the limits of logic and language. The second is more important for Wittgenstein, although he says much less about it (Stroll, 2002). Wittgenstein develops an understanding of the logical necessities that underpin scientific language. However, his main intent, emphasised in recent critical interpretation, is to show what science cannot say, and what it would never be able to say (Heaton 2000a; Stroll 2002). Indeed he concluded in the *Tractatus* that in order to understand *him,* one had to see that *his* propositions were nonsense (Wittgenstein, 1961: 6.54; Stroll, 2002).

'We feel that even when *all possible* scientific questions have been answered, the problems of life remain completely untouched. Of course there are then no questions left, and this itself is the answer' (Wittgenstein, 1961: 6.52). Wittgenstein says that only matters of fact can be put into words, and the mystical, which includes ethics and aesthetics, anything to do with value, cannot even be formulated as questions, let alone be answered.

This has implications for psychotherapy, which has been said to deal with the problems of living, or of living well. When Wittgenstein says there are no questions left that would deal with the problems of life, we deduce, as he doesn't specify, he is talking of questions to do with ultimate meaning, but also questions on what is the right way to live, how to know if 'this' is true love, how to treat other people, and so on. Neither science nor philosophy can deal with these questions, because they are not questions that admit of logical answers, however tempted we are to look for them. Elsewhere he says there are no big questions, only little ones. In his paper on ethics (Wittgenstein, 1993a), he states that one can express oneself for example by saying 'life is a miracle', and this is important ethically, but such expressions lie outside the use of language in logical propositions.

Wittgenstein's philosophy developed far beyond his initial position. It became more a method aimed at questioning the way language is used, and the false pictures of things and ourselves that we form when we speak or write unthinkingly. He thought that philosophy should be a therapy that undoes the confusion and suffering caused by mistaken ideas. He was not interested in developing a theory of persons, or of the mind. His method has considerable importance for psychiatry, psychology and psychotherapy because it offers a non-technical approach to thinking about therapeutic problems, and because it undercuts any attempt to develop a metapsychology or any theory that purports to explain the inner workings of the mind or of people. I want to emphasise this point. Wittgenstein shows how little science can ever contribute to understanding people.

One picture of the mind is of a hidden territory, with dark forces and repressed knowledge. To the psychodynamic theorist, the mind is interior, private, known only to the individual, yet paradoxically, the psychoanalyst, through his metapsychological theories, believes he knows what is really going on that the patient is unconscious of.

Gilbert Ryle, criticising psychologism generally, talks of 'the Ghost in the machine' (1949). The mind is seen as a mechanical device, similar but different to the body. While hardly new, and close to Freud's original impulse, modern neuroscience has substituted the brain, or neurogenetics, as the current all-embracing explanatory hypothesis (Bennett & Hacker, 2003).

For Wittgenstein, Heaton and others, 'the mind' or 'the self' cannot in any true sense be objects of scientific study. Wittgenstein says, 'the subject does not belong to the world, rather the subject is a limit of the world' (Wittgenstein, 1961: 5.632), and 'the I, that is what is deeply mysterious' (cited in Heaton, 2000a: 59).

That there is no object of scientific study that would correspond to 'the mind' is not immediately obvious. We can study a tree because it is there in the world to be examined in whatever way we choose. If you study enough trees you can make general statements about their structure. Yet according to Wittgenstein's notion of language games, the term 'tree' takes on its 'treeness' because of its use in a particular community of speakers. So even here there is a question about the nature of the object. Is the scientifically defined tree the essence of the tree? Or is it just the agreement of a particular school of botanists on the range of application of the term? The mind is not accessible in the same way as a tree. Yet we assume that by making certain sorts of observations we can observe the mind at work.

Einstein's metaphor for the object of physics may be helpful:

> Physical concepts are free creations of the human mind, and are not, however it may seem, uniquely determined by the external world. In our endeavour to understand reality we are somewhat like a man trying to understand the mechanism of a closed watch. He sees the face and the moving hands, even hears it ticking, but he has no way of opening the case. If he is ingenious he may form some picture of a mechanism which could be responsible for all the things which he observes, but he may never be quite sure his picture is the only one which could explain his observations. He will never be able to compare his picture with the real mechanism and he cannot even imagine the possibility of the meaning of such a comparison. (cited in Zukav, 1979: 35)

The universe, as well as the mind that explores the universe, are more complex than this metaphor suggests. Thought and matter are closely related. Think and thing are related in derivation ('now there's a thing' suggests something we are taken up with in thought) and the word 'reality' derives from the Latin words for think and thing. If we expand Einstein's metaphor to describe the study of the mind, it is like the internal stuff of the watch, if stuff it is, trying to look inside itself.

Wittgenstein cuts across this. He states that 'one of the most dangerous ideas for a philosopher is, oddly enough, that we think with our heads or in our heads. [This] idea … gives him something occult' (Heaton, 2000b: 45). Wittgenstein is clear that nothing is hidden, but we create false pictures that confuse us. Because we want to objectify everything, we imagine the mind, as Freud did, to be something like Einstein's closed watch, and we try to deduce all sorts of internal mechanisms that might explain what we take to be our observations. There are similarities between Wittgenstein's clarity that we seek these internal explanatory mechanisms at our peril, at the cost of wasted time in the desert of explanations, and the Buddhist doctrine of 'no mind'.

There are stories that demonstrate the 'no mind' from Zen Buddhism. A man seeking for enlightenment as to the true nature of his mind spent many days in the snow on a mountainside outside the cave of a known teacher. Every time he tried to enter the cave he was roughly shoved outside again. Finally the seeker cut off his left arm in frustration (no minor self-harm here!). Entering the cave carrying his arm, he said 'Master, pacify my mind.' The master said, 'Lay out your mind before me and I will pacify it.' The student attained satori, or enlightenment, at that moment (Watts, 1989).

Explanations never really capture the point, which illustrates I think Wittgenstein's insistence that there are some things, often the most important, that can be shown, but not said. The point of the 'lay out your mind before me' is that there is no thing that is the mind, nor is there a self as object which can be objectively observed. This is central to Buddhism.[1]

Another way of considering this is to think of the grammatical distinction between concrete and abstract nouns. In psychiatry and psychology we very easily confuse the two. Concrete nouns denote solid physical objects. Apples, trees, and tables are denoted by concrete nouns. Abstract nouns, such as democracy, or mind, or love, denote concepts or ideas. These don't have a concrete existence, even if we think we can see the effects they have at times. Democracy, or love, can be said to exist in that they have a force or power in human relationships, and there are social and institutional structures built around them. Buddhism has categories for things that both exist and don't exist, and for things that neither exist nor don't exist. We in the West, on the other hand, seem to get ourselves into terrible knots in trying to define the nature of ideas which have no material existence, even if they have a conceptual force, for example, mental illnesses could be said to be ideas of this sort, rather than things or entities with a material existence.

The problem of knowing about 'the mind' is similar and indeed closely related to that of knowing about language. Wittgenstein shows that there can be no overarching theory of language that can be constructed. In order to understand language and all the philosophical intricacies that arise Wittgenstein says, 'we would have to plough through the whole of language' (Wittgenstein, 1993b: 195). Each language has its own grammar, and within that there are infinite usages, sentence construction and, more importantly, meanings that can be conveyed. There are, of course, rules that govern usage and sentence construction, and these rules generally have to do with ensuring that spoken or written language makes sense. A lot of what Wittgenstein does in his later writing is to investigate how language makes sense. This is very different from looking for explanations. His

---

1. It is of note that Buddhist and Taoist ideas were discussed a lot in psychology and psychotherapy circles in the 1960s and 70s, and there is now a school of Buddhist psychotherapy. Mindfulness is used as a technique in Dialectical Behaviour Therapy. The study of 'the mind', or rather 'no mind', is at the heart of Buddhism, but Western psychology has not taken this on in great depth.

invocation is 'don't think, but look' (Wittgenstein, 1963: 66; Stroll, 2002). Heaton argues that discovering what does and doesn't make sense in one's life is most important in psychotherapy.

We live inside language, or better, we live language and language lives us. The attempt to refine scientific language or legal language into a codified, objective structure out of the complexity of lived language represents a tiny fragment of the possibilities of language even if we have come to feel that our lives are dominated by these fragments. They are, as Wittgenstein shows, language games that have a limited meaning within a limited context.

Rather than study the mind, which we can never define or pin down, Wittgenstein looks closely at how we use language and how confusions arise because we do not think about what we are saying, or because we think too much and want to be clever. Wittgenstein says, 'a picture held us captive. And we could not get outside it, for it lay in our language and language seemed to repeat it to us inexorably' (Wittgenstein, 1963: 115). Mentalism, or psychologism, the notion that events in our head are determinative and explanatory of our behaviour, is the picture that holds us captive in psychology, psychiatry and psychotherapy.[2]

Wittgenstein is not proposing that the mind is an epiphenomenon, 'the froth of consciousness', as one philosopher puts it. Considering the grammar of life is profound, and deeply challenging. It can set us free from competitive schools of therapy, each insisting that they have the truth. It may overcome the deeply confused and confusing notion of an inner world separate from an outer world, with the resulting problems of projection, introjection, and sealed off domains of the psyche, which are satisfyingly mysterious but which ultimately are blind alleys. But no theory can set us free from the struggle and the pain of existence. So often it seems that theory functions as a barrier between ourselves and the pain of life, and is likely to lead us away from 'authentic' experience, and an encounter with the other.

It is hard to get away from explanation altogether. For example, in thinking about psychoanalytic explanation, Heaton (2000a) points out that it is possible to read the stories of Freud's patients quite differently from his use of them to found his metapsychology. In imperial Vienna there was a cultural invocation preventing the discussion of sexuality. Yet Freud wanted his patients to free associate about things that led inevitably in Freud's mind to sex.

Freud gave the famous example of a mixed group of students discussing literature. A book about gladiators was mentioned. No one could remember the title, which was *Ben Hur*. *Hur* in German is whore. So Freud talks about repression of sexual material. Repression is an explanatory concept with no objective referent, just its detection in the situation by Freud. Heaton points out that we can 'explain' this in other ways, namely that in the culture of the time it was simply too embarrassing to mention the word 'whore' in polite mixed company. Freud's use of the term 'repression' disguised a socio-cultural critique, claiming instead the 'scientific discovery' of an intra-psychic mechanism.

---

2. Husserl, the founder of phenomenology, also opposed psychologism.

It takes some effort and experience of life for most people to learn a more sophisticated language than their childhood-given words and unformed concepts around sexuality. Children simply do not have sophisticated concepts or theories about sexuality (Heaton, 2000a), or indeed around the complexities of relationships generally. When someone comes to a therapist it may not be difficult for the therapist, providing she has some courage and understanding, to see the patient's confusion more clearly than he can himself. Seeing that people often don't have words, or cannot use words, may be better than saying that the patient is 'resisting' insight into 'repressed' or 'denied' thoughts and feelings. This is particularly important in dealing with people who have been abused or neglected. A major aspect of abuse is the parents' failing deliberately or otherwise to speak of the child's experience, so that they do not learn 'the words to say it'. Instead of being able to say 'I am hurt and angry' and then say why, the abused person acts in a hurt and angry way, but with other emotions, none of them recognisable, mixed in.

Heidegger has contributed to the phenomenological critique of psychology and psychiatry. Heidegger has no place for the unconscious. He prefers a notion of hesitation before the truth. Heidegger is a difficult philosopher, not least because of his albeit brief membership of the Nazi party in 1934 and his own hesitation before the truth of fascism. More particularly, those of a more positivist persuasion find him opaque, and part of some 'anti-science' trope in postmodernism. He does, for example in the *Zollikon Seminars* given to psychiatrists, draw out the limits to scientific explanation in a similar way to Wittgenstein (Heidegger, 1987). He is a profound writer on language and the problematic relationship between language and truth.

Language for Heidegger is a form of revelation. *Aletheia*, the unhidden, is allowed to stand forth when we are seized by language, and language speaks us. In contrast is the vast domain of the unspoken, the forgotten, the unrealised. *Lethe* is the river of forgetfulness we cross at death, so for Heidegger things come to life when they come to language (Heidegger, 1971). Lacan, who was influenced by Heidegger, talks of the full word in contrast to the empty word (1968). Full speech is connected both with Heidegger's notion of authenticity, and a psychoanalytic notion of connecting the signified, the hidden meaning of the symptom, with the words that bring it to a true discourse between patient and analyst. The notion of authenticity is difficult, as Heidegger realised. Without going into this in any depth, what Heidegger tries to show is that language or speech is closer to truth when it has a poetic force, when one is seized in the moment by a particular form of words, when the words leap unbidden from your mouth.[3]

Kierkegaard is another of the many philosophers who should be considered in relation to the fields that delve into the *psyche*. Kierkegaard deserves much more than a brief mention. He is considered one of the originators of a phenomenological style which approaches the problems of being human through an ever-deepening description,

---

3. Homer's Odysseus at times confesses that his words are forced out of him by his heart speaking, although usually he is very judicious and careful with what he says. Hamlet even more poignantly says, 'break my heart, for I must hold my tongue' (Act I Scene II, 363).

avoiding explanatory concepts. Description has the advantage of remaining open to scrutiny, whereas explanation in the face-to-face relationship tends to close discourse down. Kierkegaard rigorously defends subjectivity in the face of the rising tide of objectivity as the guarantee of truth and knowledge (1992).

One of Kierkegaard's famous works is *The Sickness Unto Death* (1980), which is about despair. Despair is much more than depression, and could hardly be a diagnostic category, as we all suffer from despair, and those who don't realise it are in greater despair than those who do. Kierkegaard's descriptions of the varieties of despair encompass many of the rather empty ways that people lead their lives. Many people who come into psychotherapy feeling at a loss, their lives meaningless, are recognisably in despair. Kierkegaard's description of demonic despair fits many patients who have been abused and who almost delight in the furious destruction that runs through their lives:

> Demonic despair is the most intensive form of the despair: in despair to will to be oneself ... In hatred towards existence, it wills to be itself, wills to be itself in accordance with its misery. Not even in defiance does it will to be itself, but for spite: not even in defiance does it want to tear itself loose from the power that established it, but for spite wants to force itself upon it, to obtrude defiantly upon it, wants to adhere to it out of malice ... Rebelling against all existence, [she] feels that [she] has obtained evidence against it, against its goodness. The person in despair believes that she herself is the evidence, and that is what she wants to be ... herself in her torment. (Kierkegaard, 1980: 73)

Kierkegaard here shows the power of language and 'ordinary' (meaning non-theoretical) description. It is hard to imagine a more precise account of the battle that some of those locked into self-harm and other self-destructive actions carry on primarily with themselves as well as with those who try to care for them.

THE IMPORTANCE OF ETHICS

Ethics, although often talked of in this way, is not a separate domain. All human action can be judged on an ethical dimension, although we probably don't do this most of the time. Spontaneous action might be said to inhabit ethics, just as people inhabit language, even if most actions don't call up much of an ethical dilemma. In other words we mostly act without thinking as we go whether we are being ethical or not. In this sense the frame of our action is 'unconscious' (although not in the Freudian sense), whether it is speech or another sort of action. It is not that we cannot be aware of it, only that it is not intentionally called to mind for most ordinary actions.

For more formal purposes we do crystallise the ethical dimension into a code or law or set of rules, and most societies or organisations depend on this. Increasingly everything we do is governed by policies, protocols and procedures. This formalising of human action is of a very different order from a spontaneous, lived ethics that is implicit rather than explicit.

Wittgenstein, as mentioned above, attempted to demonstrate that ethics cannot be founded in logical propositions and therefore cannot be founded scientifically (1993). Ethics, he says, derives from a 'temptation' to make absolute statements. Absolute statements are always logically nonsense even though they may be deeply profound. 'I feel that this world is absolutely marvellous' is an example Wittgenstein uses. As a proposition it is meaningless because it is capable neither of proof nor refutation. Wittgenstein thought such speech was highly important, but it is 'an expression by means of language', not a 'logical proposition in language'.

Implicit in this expression: 'I feel that this world is absolutely marvellous', is a relationship to the world, to oneself, and to other people. For Wittgenstein ethics are founded in this sense or experience that existence is miraculous. He thought that this must be allowed as the basis of ethics even though it can never be dealt with by logic or by science.

When it comes to dealing with patients, or clients, practice must remain a practice, so something fallible, but also something that develops, that broadens or deepens with experience. Much that is done in medicine and psychotherapy is prescribed, set within guidelines, informed by protocols or the National Service Framework. Clearly the intention of these guidelines is to ensure best practice is carried out everywhere, in a democratically and equally resourced NHS. This seems ethical, but this is a deeper issue. It is only fair, we might say, that if everybody pays taxes, the benefit of these taxes should be available to everyone. But fairness is not the only determinant of ethics.

It is commonplace in guidelines in medicine that each person is to be treated as an individual. The GMC asks this of doctors. Against this is the old problem of 'the kidney in bed 6', the busy physician's or surgeon's reduction of the individual to the diagnosis. Whatever the branch of medicine there is always the temptation to treat 'x' as just another instance of his or her illness. This may be inadvertently encouraged by the culture of National Institute for Health and Clinical Excellence (NICE) guidelines and evidence-based medicine, which, in demanding the best treatment for everyone, prescribes the same treatment for everyone with a particular condition. Of course it is hard to deny the validity of guidelines in many situations—if I need a knee replacement I want it done in the best way, and I want my new knee to be as good as yours. In therapy this may be more problematic, even if there is evidence that CBT is as effective as antidepressants for many cases of depression.

People are very sensitive to being treated as 'just another one', although it should not be impossible to combine protocol-based treatment with attunement to the individual person. 'Conveyer belt' is a common expression people use when being wheeled through a system as a case of whatever. This may be not so bad if you have a 'deserving' illness such as a heart attack, provided you are a non-smoker! If you are 'undeserving', say with a self-inflicted injury, dirty looks and muttered derogatory labels like 'another borderline' are more likely.

While it may not require a particular ethical stance in psychotherapy to avoid falling back on a diagnosis and just apply the appropriate technique (being 'natural' with a client comes naturally at least to some practitioners), I am arguing that it may be that attention to the individual person and her story is what is most therapeutic. We may argue that the personal aspects of the treatment are the frame of what happens (respect, careful listening, non-discrimination) when the technique is applied, but it still is a different thing when the therapy itself is radically directed at the person, not her 'condition'.

What I am interested in here is how this understanding of ethics can inform psychiatry, psychology and the practice of psychotherapy. I am not saying that we don't need an ethical frame or a code of ethics. But the ethical dimension is much more than a code to be applied in a legalistic manner when there is a complaint or malpractice.

Berger's book, *A Fortunate Man* (2005), emphasises the relationship between doctor and patient, and the implication of the doctor in that relationship. The doctor is hero, saviour, wise counsellor, privileged member of the community, or omnipresent servant of the community without privacy or her own needs. How the doctor acts into these fantastic roles relates to her personal qualities, the likelihood of burnout or depression, and the quality of care. Perhaps more importantly, descriptions of practice like this offer a different sort of evidence to more 'objective' studies that only measure outcomes in the patient or audit service delivery. Similarly, a recent *Journal of the Royal Society of Medicine* has a series of articles on the doctor as a human being, and the interpersonal relationships that are always prior to and implicit in the more technical aspects of medical practice. These provide a counter strand of evidence to institutions like the Healthcare Commission and the NICE guidelines which seem to reduce medical practice to the following of policies and protocols.

The point here is that the ethical relationship is not one that can be reduced to a set of rules, nor can it be put into a protocol. It is something else, to do with what Heaton (2000b) has called style. Heaton has discussed this particularly in relation to the charismatic R.D. Laing, who was one of the main founders of the Philadelphia Association. It would be absurd to suggest that we should be like Laing, who had a very destructive side to his charisma. However we can all have style, hopefully in the sense of how one engages with the patient or client, how one brings oneself into the room, and overcomes shyness as Berger's doctor had to, or overcomes all sorts of other personal difficulties when facing the patient. This is only partly to do with how one is a professional, which is informed by some basic ethical rules, such as the Hippocratic Oath. The style of the professional is not simply personal, or fashionable, but has to do with taking up a stance, or a position, with authorising oneself albeit within a tradition. These comments do not have any finality to them, and are sketchy. I can only suggest a few pointers. But it is an area that is perhaps being recognised again, paradoxically as professional practice is increasingly regulated and scrutinised.

THE POSSIBILITIES AND LIMITS
OF THERAPEUTIC LANGUAGE

Therapy is not concerned with the mind, nor an imagined interiority. Therapy is not concerned with theoretical explanations of how the mind works. So therapy is not about explaining the patient to herself in any scientific or pseudo-scientific way. Therapy is concerned with the person in her particularity, in her entanglements with others, and her relationship with herself, and may best occur in a relationship with another who has some understanding with the struggles of living. It involves speech, and before someone can speak there must be someone who is listening (Fiumara, 1990).

I want to return to our starting point: 'Philosophy ... leaves everything as it is' (Wittgenstein, 1993b: 49). Wittgenstein also states: 'we cannot terminate a disease of thought ... slow cure is all important.' These two statements in part contradict each other, but have a certain kinship. The reason I want to repeat 'philosophy changes nothing' is not to be nihilistic, but to emphasise the ethical and practical position implied. Freud said that the curative aspect of psychoanalysis was incidental and that it was the scientific, investigative aspect that was to be furthered by close work with the patient. Although I disagree with Freud that it has anything to do with science, there is something about this getting in close, and the spirit of enquiry, that is important. It is in a sense trying to lay everything out, even trying to make a clear diagnosis, although not exactly in the medical sense. It is starting where the patient is and allowing them to set the pace. Often as therapists we feel we ought to be able to change things for the patient, and the quicker the better.

Wittgenstein says one of the greatest impediments to philosophy is the expectation of new, deep, or unheard-of elucidations. We can say the same of psychotherapy. What can happen, say with very disturbed patients, which an analyst would call countertransference, is our wish for a magical answer to a problem we are stuck in. Or we simply want to get out of the awful situation, out of the room with the hopelessly frozen patient, whom at that moment we hate, but our professional obligation dictates that we do it kindly, and with something for the patient. As a psychologist colleague once said, in working with some patients one is left, stripped bare of everything, including professional training, and one's sense of having anything to offer.

Berger says that the key in the doctor–patient relationship is recognition. 'The doctor, in order to recognize the illness fully ... must first recognise the patient as a person' (Berger, 2005: 68).

> An unhappy man comes to a doctor to offer him an illness, in the hope that this part of him at least is recognizable. His proper self he believes to be unknowable. In the light of the world he is nobody; by his own lights the world is nothing ... If the man can begin to feel recognized—and such recognition may well include aspects of his character which he has not yet recognized himself—the hopeless nature of his unhappiness will have been changed. (Berger, 2005: 70)

Of a physical illness Berger says, 'patients are inordinately relieved when doctors give their complaint a name. The name may mean very little to them ... but because it has a name, it has an independent existence from them' (ibid.: 74).

Compare this with Wittgenstein: 'The philosopher strives to find the liberating word, that is, the word that finally permits us to grasp what up until now has intangibly weighed down our consciousness.' And again, 'the philosopher delivers the word to us with which [we] can express the thing and render it harmless' (Wittgenstein, 1993b: 165).

Berger's idea is that naming an illness is an important step in relieving the patient's nameless dread, and the threat that is part of the patient's very being. There are several things here. First, the patient is relieved by the naming of the illness, because it brings the mystery of his unwellness into the known world. It may confirm or relieve the patient of his worst fears, but it also shows the patient that someone understands his condition, and may be able to give further relief. A traditional shaman does something similar within that particular culture. In this the authority of the doctor is important. Second, something related but different happens in psychotherapy. Recognition is still the basis, but the recognition of the patient's 'heart of darkness' is done in such a way that the power to intervene largely remains with the patient. This is fundamental to 'psychoanalytic' therapies, whereas in therapies such as CBT the therapist remains more in charge of the interventions, even if the patient has to take them on and do homework. Third, and with a somewhat different intention, naming the illness helps to separate it from the patient's identity. Mental illness tends to be different in this sense from physical illness—one *is* a schizophrenic or an anorexic, whereas one *has* pneumonia, or multiple sclerosis. 'Externalising' the illness, as with anorexia, may help the young person especially fight something that does at times seem to have a life of its own.

I do not want to suggest that psychotherapy is only about naming the problem. Rather, as Heaton (2000a) suggests, psychotherapeutic language is about making sense of what the patient says, in terms both patient and therapist understand. It is therefore, as I've said, something both are involved in; the therapist is not at one remove, observing the patient. The therapist listens to enable the patient to speak, and although hopefully not caught up in the knot in the same way as the patient, nevertheless is interested in the sense that Heidegger suggests, which is to be in amongst it (*inter esse*).

Language cannot in any simple sense explain things away. Language cannot change how things are, but recognition of one's state may sometimes be enlightening. Lacan says that language in the form of interpretation cannot reduce the transference (Lacan, 1968). The terms 'transference' and 'counter-transference' are, I think, confusing, implying as they do that the feelings arising in the therapeutic relationship come from elsewhere. It is true that the emotions and associated behaviours that a patient brings to treatment have arisen prior to the therapeutic relationship. But now they come up here in this relationship. And things the therapist does may be mistaken, or may make the patient angry for very good reasons. The point is that we are always implicated in the relationship, which is what makes it so difficult, and why a thorough training is so important. The training is not to give you theoretical knowledge so you always know where you are in the relationship, but to help you survive uncertainty and the terror of the face to face.

CONCLUSIONS

I have argued here that the mind does not exist as an entity that allows scientific study, which is not to say that brain function, or aspects such as memory or language can't be studied, as long as this is not seen as the mind. Most importantly, scientific study of how brains work is very different from getting to know people or patients, and this is at the heart of the ethical question. Even if notions of individuality mislead us as to the extent of the differences between us, there is no substitute for careful attention and listening to the other's story as the foundation of ethical practice. This is not and never will be something we elucidate through science.

Wittgenstein thought philosophy could provide a therapeutic method that did not depend on a theory of the mind. He is interested primarily in the way we use language and how we get confused and captured by our 'grammar'. He also makes it clear that the most difficult thing is to undo the false pictures we live by. Simple logical argument is to no avail, as we see with a young girl who is saying 'I am fat' while being quite the opposite. While CBT and various other therapeutic methods offer techniques that may attempt to undo this thought, or other thoughts such as, 'my life is worthless, I do not deserve to live, so I will kill myself', the limits are easily reached, especially if we deal with what tend to get called 'complex cases'. What is often striking when talking to a patient on these subjects is how limited the conversation is. In order to have something to talk about you have to change the subject.

How do we produce change? Wittgenstein says, 'We cannot say that everything flows. That everything flows must lie in how language touches reality' (Wittgenstein, 1993: 189). What Wittgenstein means here is difficult. When our words flow freely things constantly move on; in psychotherapy that is 'flowing', things will move on. Often our attempts to change things deliberately and in a planned way are false—we cannot force things to move. Language by its nature participates in change, but language does not change things as an active force. Or at least a poem, a song, a film, a novel, have as much chance of changing the world, or a person, as any of our planned cognitive or psychoanalytic interventions. This goes against the positivism of the age, and the evidence base is not likely to get to this kind of understanding. Is it possible that philosophy can change some things?

REFERENCES

Bennett, MR & Hacker, PMS (2003) *Philosophical Foundations of Neuroscience*. Oxford: Blackwell.

Berger, J (2005) *A Fortunate Man: The story of a country doctor*. London: Royal College of General Practitioners.

Fiumara, GC (1990) *The Other Side of Language: A philosophy of listening* (C Lambert, Trans). London: Routledge.

Heaton, J (2000a) On RD Laing: Style, sorcery, alienation. *Psychoanalytic Review, 87* (4), 511–26.

Heaton, J (2000b) *Wittgenstein and Psychoanalysis*. Cambridge: Icon Books.
Heidegger, M (1971) *On the Way to Language*. San Francisco, CA: Harper & Row.
Heidegger, M (1987) *Zollikon Seminars,* M Boss (Ed). Evanston, IL: Northwestern University Press.
Kierkegaard, S (1980) *The Sickness unto Death* (HV Hong & EH Hong, Trans). Princeton, NJ: Princeton University Press.
Kierkegaard, S (1992) *Concluding Unscientific Postscript to Philosophical Fragments* (HV Hong & EH Hong, Trans). Princeton, NJ: Princeton University Press.
Lacan, J (1968) *Speech and Language in Psychoanalysis* (A Wilden, Trans). Baltimore, MD/London: John Hopkins University Press.
Ryle, G (1949) *The Concept of Mind*. Harmondsworth: Penguin.
Stroll, A (2002) *Wittgenstein*. Oxford: Oneworld.
Watts, A (1989) *The Way of Zen*. New York: Vintage.
Wittgenstein, L (1953) *Philosophical Investigations,* GEM Anscombe & R Rhees (Eds), (GEM Anscombe, Trans). Oxford: Blackwell.
Wittgenstein, L (1961) *Tractatus Logico-Philosophicus* (DF Pears & BF McGuiness, Trans). London: Routledge & Kegan Paul.
Wittgenstein, L (1993a) A lecture on ethics. In J Klagge & A Nordmann (Eds) *Philosophical Occasions 1912–1951* (pp 36–44). Indianapolis, IN/Cambridge: Hackett.
Wittgenstein, L (1993b) Philosophy. In J Klagge & A Nordmann (Eds) *Philosophical Occasions 1912–1951* (pp 160–99). Indianapolis, IN/Cambridge: Hackett.
Zukav, G (1979) *The Dancing Wu Li Masters: An overview of the new physics*. London: Rider.

CHAPTER 6

THE RADICAL PSYCHIATRIST AS TRICKSTER

HELEN SPANDLER

INTRODUCTION

Psychiatric practice is dependent on particular social, cultural and moral judgements about the ways in which individuals grapple with 'being human' (Jenner et al, 1993). This is one reason why it is important to develop and defend spaces in which psychiatric judgement and practice can not only be contested and challenged, but also where we can seek more genuine forms of open dialogue with, and about, 'madness', to ensure we move towards greater forms of democratic engagement and practice. However, there is always a push to close down these spaces and insist upon closure of debate and routinised practice. For example, attempts at greater democracy in mental health services and experimental 'anti-psychiatric' initiatives have often been written off as 'radical failure' (Spandler, 2006).

Drawing on recent attempts to utilise the notion of the 'trickster' as a positive force in challenging health and social care practices (e.g. White, 2006), this chapter explores how tensions and contradictions in the mental health system might be creatively explored. I argue that cultivating a 'trickster sensibility' is one way of ensuring that the conflicts, uncertainties and ambiguities, inherent in both decisions about mental health care *and* stories about radical innovations, are foregrounded in our discussions. This could help ensure that such discussions are not artificially and prematurely closed down.

I use the idea of the 'trickster' in three related ways. First, to refer to ways in which dominant psychiatric discourses and practices have been challenged *by* particular trickster-like figures, especially psychiatrists themselves. Second, to refer to the ways in which particular stories or narratives *about* tricksters circulate in particular social contexts to describe or explain a series of real or imagined historical events, as *radical failure*. Finally, I introduce a third way of viewing the creative potential of the trickster in the modern context. This explores the idea of a 'trickster politics of tensions', a politics that is not dependent upon the limitations of individual charismatic figures, but is developed and suffused through various 'paradoxical social spaces' (Rose, 1993). As a vehicle to explore these issues, I draw on the history of Paddington Day Hospital, a libertarian therapeutic community in west London (Spandler, 2006). The history of Paddington Day Hospital, and its legacy in *Asylum to Anarchy* (Baron, 1987), might be regarded as a quintessential 'trickster story' in mental health.

THE RADICAL PSYCHIATRIST AS TRICKSTER

Some commentators have, at least in passing, described radical psychiatrists, like R.D. Laing, as 'tricksters' (Burston, 1996; Doty & Hynes, 1993; Mezan, 1972; Hynes & Doty, 1993).[1] However, the potentiality of this concept in illustrating some of the opportunities and limitations of such figures in the psychiatric field has not been explored in any detail. Moreover, although the idea of the 'trickster healer' has been briefly alluded to as a possible way of viewing the role of spontaneity and mischievousness of the psychotherapist in gestalt psychotherapy, the focus was on the potential individual therapeutic value of their character and responses, rather than their wider social or cultural impact (Zimberoff & Hartman, 2003; Kopp, 1976).

The trickster is a figure from world mythology (Hyde, 1998). It is a contradictory force, both constructive and destructive, a figure that challenges dominant thinking and social conventions. On a positive level it can be an agent of change and renewal, forcing us to confront unpalatable truths, raising awkward questions and challenging our conceptions of normality and acceptability. On the flip side, this maverick figure can produce unpleasant and shocking effects, and can be experienced as destructive. The trickster is a figure that embodies and acts out various social tensions, pushing the limits of what is both possible and desirable, often through subversion and humour. The trickster can be seen as 'the mythic embodiment of ambiguity and ambivalence, doubleness and duplicity, contradiction and paradox' (Hyde, 1998: 7).

Radical psychiatrists have often either been romanticised as heroic counter-leaders or demonised and psychopathologised (Leitner, 1999; Mosher, 1991; Burston, 1996). Whilst there are many exceptions to this, I argue that the notion of the trickster is a particularly useful concept for understanding the role and impact of the radical psychiatrist, precisely because it draws our attention to their paradoxical role.[2] Moreover, unlike some commentators who have argued that the trickster represents an important but *primitive* or *infantile* stage in human evolution in terms of cultural and individual development (see for example, Jung, 1955; Radin, 1955), I argue that the paradoxical nature of the trickster means that it has both positive and negative effects in the world. It important to note that the 'trickster' is an abstraction. Actual embodied individuals are always more complex than the archetype (Hyde, 1998). I am not necessarily arguing that particular characters were *in fact* tricksters, rather that there are particular historical moments which specifically created spaces for trickster-type practices to emerge through

---

1. Incidentally, Laing himself apparently made reference to the importance of 'trickster stories' in facilitating his understanding of 'schizophrenia' (Hynes & Doty, 1993).
2. The therapeutic community movement utilised the notion of the 'charismatic leader' as a way to explain the key role of the Medical Director or Psychiatrist in developing and shaping an egalitarian and collectivist therapeutic community practice which is often at odds with the surrounding psychiatric and social culture. This notion of 'charismatic leadership' is also useful because it recognises the positive and negative consequences of such leadership on the survival of such communities (Kennard, 1991; Hobson, 1979). The idea of the trickster I discuss here could be used to complement such ideas.

the behaviour of particular individuals. These individuals, by virtue of their being sufficiently inside *and* outside the dominant psychiatric culture, were able to express this sensibility at particular times. Neither do I want to make the claim that archetypes such as the trickster necessarily represent something transcendental and universal in the human psyche (Radin, 1955; Jung, 1955). Whilst recent commentators (e.g. Hynes & Doty, 1993) have explored wide-ranging *cultural manifestations* of trickster figures, rather then their origins or essence, I want to explore their social manifestations within the specific context of psychiatric practice.

Whilst the trickster belongs to the periphery and is thus usually a marginal figure, one of the paradoxes of the trickster figure is that they require some power and influence on the 'inside' in order to have sufficient space to be able to exercise their trickster-like qualities, and to have an impact (Hyde, 1998). In this context it is worth noting that probably the most sustained and rigorous attack on the foundations of the psychiatric profession has risen from within its ranks, through the work of the psychiatrist Thomas Szasz, especially through his 'myth of mental illness' thesis (Cresswell, 2008). The social situation usually occupied by the trickster might be one of the reasons why they are usually portrayed as male figures.[3] Moreover, trickster archetypes tend to emerge in patriarchal mythologies, where the 'prime actors, even at the margins, are male' (Hyde, 1998: 8). It could be argued that the medical establishment has traditionally been male-dominated and more generally and historically, women have had a lot less actual 'freedom of movement' than men. It is precisely this quality that is a necessary defining character of the trickster who requires sufficient space, status and command to be taken seriously (Tannen, 2007). Similarly, this might also help us to understand how male *psychiatrists* have often occupied this role, at least in particular historical contexts, due to their position as simultaneously on the *inside* (of the medical profession) yet on the *outside,* by virtue of their contrary ideas and identification with seeking to make sense of the ultimate experience of exclusion (madness).

Whilst there probably has always been resistance to psychiatric practice ever since its inception (Crossley, 1999; Campbell, 1996), it wasn't until the late 1960s and early 1970s that we witnessed a sustained period of psychiatric contestation. It is often said that tricksters appear at key points of growth and change in society and represent future possibilities (Hynes & Doty, 1993). This period was beginning to see changes in the psychiatric arena itself. For example, growing unease at psychiatric hospital practice and emerging critiques of institutionalisation (e.g. Goffman, 1961) helped to energise the re-emergence of therapeutic communities as radical alternatives to the mental health system. These changes took place within a wider context of high employment and increasing demands for labour which may have spawned a new therapeutic optimism and a renewed interest in social rehabilitative psychiatry (Warner, 1994). This period

---

3. Some have argued that the trickster could be an androgynous figure as s/he might be able to transcend the boundaries between male and female. In a recent Jungian feminist account it is argued that postmodernism has enabled the development of female tricksters figures (Tannen, 2007). Nevertheless, unfortunately, as Hyde has argued, the typical trickster, at least in our cultural imagination, remains male (Hyde, 1998).

was also characterised by a heightened *political* as well as *therapeutic* optimism and activism, in the aftermath of 1968 (Brown & Hanvey, 1987).

The rise of new social movements, especially the 'New Left' and the women's liberation movement brought to the fore issues of identity, subjectivity, freedom and oppression and this made the politicisation of the field of mental health and psychiatry increasingly possible (Crossley, 1999). The convergence of progressive social forces and radicalised individuals combined with an emergence of new ideas and organisations (Freeman, 1999). The impact of wider social innovations and prefigurative practices that were developed from within the social movements were often taken up in the mental health field. For example, the emerging counter-culture supported communal living, social experimentation and innovation and this helped enable a greater toleration of madness or psychological disturbance (Crossley, 1999; Spandler, 2006). It also provided the context for greater attempts to understand distress within its wider social context. For example, perhaps the ultimate 'anti-psychiatrist'[4] and trickster, David Cooper, succinctly argued that 'madness is the expression of social contradictions against which we must struggle as such' (Cooper, 1978: 166). In typical trickster fashion, the 'anti-psychiatrists' drew our collective attention to the reality of these social conflicts (Makarius, 1993).

Therefore, the social context in this period was ripe for the emergence of trickster figures who helped bring into question certain widely held assumptions about madness and psychiatry. The lack of an organised patients' movement meant that challenge often came from within the ranks of psychiatrists and mental health professionals themselves. Such figures had sufficient power and status to challenge the role of psychiatry in social control and regulation from *within* (Crossley, 1998). Thus, despite the paradox of *psychiatrists* actively challenging psychiatric assumptions and pursuing the acceptability and intelligibility of madness, it was precisely their role *as* psychiatrists that allowed them some freedom to experiment with new ideas and practices, a freedom rarely afforded to other professionals (or non-professionals).

As the social movement theorist Alberto Melucci[5] argues, such figures often play an important part in the development of social movements by picking up and embodying a number of emerging contradictions and tensions in the social world. Contemporary social movements 'move in to occupy an intermediate space of social life where individual needs and the pressures of political innovation mesh' (Melucci, 1994: 102). These pressures or conflicts and contradictions in the social world are 'carried forward by temporary actors who bring to light the crucial dilemmas of a society' (ibid). Such figures personally occupy and command social spaces available for social innovation. However, in creating the conditions for social change and making challenges which rub against the grain of acceptable practice and ideas, they create resistance and controversy.

---

4. It was Cooper who, after all, coined the term 'anti-psychiatrist' and was probably the only radical psychiatrist to have actually identified themselves with it (Cooper, 1967).
5. Whilst Melucci used the term 'innovative counterleaders' (Melucci, 1996: 338) it could equally apply to the trickster figure.

JULIAN GOODBURN AS TRICKSTER

In this section I use some examples from my research into Paddington Day Hospital, and Julian Goodburn in particular, to demonstrate some of the features that have been attributed to trickster figures (see Hyde, 1998; White, 2006). This study offers us a unique, but lesser-known, example of the trickster and associated trickster mythologies. Goodburn was the Medical Director in charge of Paddington Day Hospital during the early 1970s. A conventionally trained psychiatrist and psychoanalyst who tried to develop a more informal, egalitarian and libertarian approach to practice. He had little contact with the famous 'anti-psychiatry' figures like R.D. Laing and David Cooper, although he was often associated with them because of his increasingly radicalised thinking and ideas.

Paddington Day Hospital was an important communicational 'node' in the UK radical psychiatric community (Spandler, 2006). It operated as a 'space of convergence' (Routledge, 2001) of various progressive counter-cultural forces that were a feature of the period, bringing together radical mental health workers who were attracted to therapeutic communities as an alterative to the conventional psychiatric hospital, ideas of anti-psychiatry, and key figures in the emerging patients' movement. As a result, Paddington Day Hospital offered a rich context for innovation.

The trickster reminds us that we need to question our underlying assumptions, rules and values about what is right and wrong; they ultimately 'shake up' our thinking (White, 2006). There are a number of examples of Goodburn's role in challenging accepted psychiatric, psychoanalytic *and* therapeutic community thinking at the day hospital. He not only challenged the ideologies of the prevailing 'psy' professions but he also challenged patients' own perceptions of themselves in relation to the world and their place within it. Rather than seeing individuals as victims of 'mental illness', like the other 'anti-psychiatrists', Goodburn saw patients as carriers of wider social tensions:

> There is a correlation between the contradiction, or disquiet that they're experiencing, and the contradiction or disquiet that everybody ought to be experiencing a propos some factor of society at large, which, you know, they are, through circumstances of their particular experience, the bearer of—the victim of, you might even say—and will subsequently manifest this as if it were something solely going on in them, when in fact it is going on in them, but as a consequence of the fact that these issues are not resolved in the world at large, and it just happens that they are the person standing on that particular street corner at that particular time who've copped it, as it were. (Goodburn, cited in Spandler, 2006: 33)[6]

---

6. It is possible to apply similar logic to the situation of the trickster or radical innovator. In other words, a particular constellation of social, cultural and personal forces is required to radicalise the psychiatrist at this time, such that they become potential innovators i.e. it is not purely a matter of historical inevitability or personal psychology (or pathology).

He challenged the notion of the role of the Medical Director (the consultant psychiatrist) in a psychiatric setting by refusing to take 'medical' responsibility for the day hospital and carry out official mental health assessments, give out diagnoses, hand out palliatives or sign their medical certificates which would designate patients as 'mentally ill'. Not wanting to perpetuate their role as helpless victims and as 'mental patients', staff challenged their need to be designated 'sick'. As a result the staff queried the need to sign medical certificates. Goodburn had a confrontational therapy style, pushing issues to their limits in an attempt to force personal and political awareness. Some of this style was developed from his long-time association with the group psychoanalyst, Henry Ezriel, although Goodburn radicalised Ezriel's approach in the more politically aware context of the day hospital, following a politicised campaign to save it from closure.

Humour was an important and often under-recognised trait of both Ezriel and Goodburn, who presented their ideas and experiences with case studies, stories and self-mocking jokes (Thomas, 2002). However, despite the difficulty of relaying the potency of humour in text, humour is a crucial feature of the trickster. Goodburn used psychoanalytic interpretation and humour in an attempt to reveal underlying interpersonal, social and political dynamics which were impacting on the situation at Paddington, in what could be considered as a form of 'metaplay' engaged in by the trickster. Metaplay is a sort of 'inversionary logic that probes and disassembles the most serious rules of "normal" social behaviour, or the behaviour expected of a person in a particular role or position' (Hynes, 1993: 30). On one occasion Goodburn was reported as being found under a table refusing to make decisions on behalf of the patients, forcing them to take responsibility for their own lives and actions; on another occasion as barricaded into one of the therapy group rooms for refusing to sign patients' medical certificates (Spandler, 2001).

The trickster also reminds us that we actively participate in the shaping of this world and challenges the prevailing belief that any social order is absolute, objective and unchallengeable (Hynes, 1993; Hyde, 1998). Goodburn wanted to allow the day hospital patients to develop their own freedom without external constraints and was intent on trying to create the best conditions through which people could take charge and shape the world as they saw fit, by challenging their notions of themselves as sick or in need of external leadership:

> We desperately need a religion, a belief system, a sense of being overburdened, overpowered, oppressed with it, in order to lull our anxiety that we're actually in a position to take charge of the situation, and shape it as we see fit.
> (Goodburn, cited in Spandler, 2002: 136)

Distinctions between the 'outside' and the 'inside' and the 'mentally well' and 'ill' were frequently put to question, not only by Goodburn, but by patients and staff at the day hospital. For example, the power structure of the day hospital and the distinctions between patients and staff were often questioned. Questions were asked such as 'why are the staff paid salaries while the patients have to survive on social security?' (Durkin,

1972: 14). In addition, Goodburn tried to give keys to patients of the day hospital and record proceedings of the official inquiry which proceeded into the functioning of the day hospital, so patients could know what was going on. Although both of these attempts were thwarted (and condemned) it was illustrative of the ways in which the boundaries of acceptability were continually questioned.

The trickster actively 'troubles' accepted and comfortable distinctions and boundaries (Hyde, 1998). Goodburn challenged many of the accepted boundaries of traditional psychoanalytic and psychiatric practice, for example by experimenting with turning the day hospital into one 'large group' session through which personal, institutional and political processes could be reflected upon. His position within a therapeutic community setting, with its emphasis on shared collective understandings, democratisation and 'cultures of enquiry' (Norton, 1996) enabled opportunities for the trickster to 'create lively talk where there has been silence', 'speak fresh' and 'tickle the imaginations of his kinsfolk' (White, 2006: 36).

> Reflective practitioners need to tell stories about themselves and others ... that defend the openness of human conversation and raise possibilities that *things could be otherwise*—not because they necessarily *ought* to be, but so that they *might* be. (White, 2006: 27)

In this context, the trickster is able to expand the realm of thinking possibilities which, in turn, allows the space behind them to expand (at least for a while). For example, the libertarianism fostered by Goodburn and his colleagues at Paddington contributed to the conditions in which the mental patients' unions (MPU), the first network of organised patients' groups in the UK, were able to form.[7] Although it cannot be argued that Paddington or Goodburn played an active part in the development of the MPU, the early MPU activists clearly felt that Goodburn's libertarianism was practically as well as theoretically important, for example one activist pointed out that 'without his opening the doors we would never actually have met' (Douieb, cited in Spandler, 2006: 58).

LIMITATIONS OF THE PSYCHIATRIST AS TRICKSTER

Whilst the radical psychiatrist as trickster can be seen as a positive force for change in contributing to emerging radical mental health movements, it inevitably expresses a number of limitations and problems. Indeed, radical psychiatrists occupy a 'paradoxical space' in which they simultaneously subvert, and yet often also reproduce, prevailing power relations. In other words, as the actual embodiment of paradox, the trickster psychiatrist often reproduces the very contradictions they reveal, precisely because of their inside/outside status. The contradictions that the radical psychiatrist exposes are

---

7. It is important to recognise that other mental patients' unions were forming around this time (the Scottish Union of Mental Patients was probably the first). However, the national network of patients' unions in England really took off following a meeting at Paddington Day Hospital in 1973.

often merely mirrored back through their actions, rather than ultimately challenged. For example, some have argued that the domination of therapeutic communities by psychiatrists, however well-meaning, ultimately limits the progress and innovation of alternative community practices (Haddon, 1979). This is the limitation of the trickster; if 'it only mirrors the thing it opposes, it discovers no secret passage into new worlds' (Hyde, 1998: 271).

In addition, tricksters can become so *marked* by what they oppose, that their challenges often fold back on themselves and become part of the problem (Parker et al, 1995). In part, this is because, as Audre Lorde famously put it, 'the master's tools will never dismantle the master's house' (Lorde, 2000). In other words, even though the radical psychiatrists frequently used 'alternative' psychiatric discourse, they ultimately had more power to do so than patients, or other workers. Their 'alternative' could still be considered in the broader lexicon of the 'psy' disciplines, which tries to impose particular forms of expert psychological knowledge (Miller & Rose, 1986).

For example, Goodburn's use of psychoanalytic understandings both provided important insights into the dynamics within and beyond the day hospital, but was also experienced by many as not only limited, but also oppressive. Some patients and staff viewed psychoanalytic interpretation as being wielded round as a new regime of psychological truth, however seemingly democratic (Baron, 1987). Indeed, one of the dangers of the trickster's subversive use of humour is the possibility of offending or humiliating others. Baron's book is littered with many possible examples of this, for instance, what appear to be far-fetched and mocking interpretations of patients' motives. This is one way in which the trickster is seen as walking a fine line between creativity and destructiveness (Hynes & Doty, 1993).[8]

Furthermore, whilst boundary crossing and subversion may be a necessary condition for creating challenging 'lively talk', it is not sufficient. Moreover, it often excludes others (White, 2006). For example, it appeared that many women patients felt considerably less safe within the informal and libertarian atmosphere at Paddington (Baron, 1987; Spandler, 2006).

Similarly, many feminists have criticised the anti-psychiatrists for their disregard of sexual politics and, as a result, reproducing gender inequalities in their practice (Burstow, 2005; Showalter, 1987). Indeed the 'tyranny of structurelessness' became a well-known (feminist) critique of much libertarian organising, which often left the oppressed and powerless even more silenced and marginalised, through unacknowledged power structures (Freeman, 1974/1984). In addition, whilst such charismatic figures may prove inspirational in provoking challenges which form the basis of initiatives that welcome change, uncertainty and risk (Alaszewski, Manthorpe & Walsh, 1995), they are less adept at providing the security, support and sustainability that such initiatives require (Hinshelwood, 1987).

The lack of serious attention to power relationships and dynamics, especially race and gender, was an important critique of anti-psychiatric alternatives more generally

---

8. This tension is summed up by the subtitle of Mullan's edited collection of commentaries about Laing: *RD Laing: Creative destroyer* (Mullan, 1997).

(Showalter, 1987; Parker et al, 1995). Of course, the more obvious point that the radical psychiatrists tended to be white, middle class and male can be been seen as limiting their effectiveness as social innovators. It could also be argued that dissent *within* the ranks is a more acceptable form of protest and can be more effectively co-opted and contained. In this way, threats can be more successfully reincorporated, not least because the challenge doesn't threaten other, more fundamental, aspects of the status quo.[9]

In sum, the concept of the trickster is useful because it recognises both the possibilities and limitations of the radical psychiatrist as an 'agent provocateur' within psychiatry. The limitations outlined here draw attention to the paradox at the heart of the subversive trickster figure, that in breaking the rules, they confirm the rules (Hynes & Doty, 1993). That the history of Paddington Day Hospital was so clearly riddled with these tensions and paradoxes marks it as an important moment in history. Not only did patients and staff struggle to collectively defend the progressive elements of the day hospital, they were also vociferous in resisting its practices when it failed to meet their expectations. However, rather than the history of Paddington Day Hospital being seen as an important lesson in revealing and reflecting on these tensions, it became a 'trickster story' *par excellence*, through Claire Baron's highly influential book *Asylum to Anarchy* (Baron, 1987).

TRICKSTER STORIES OF RADICAL FAILURE

Asylum to Anarchy is a well-known, influential and anonymised account of Paddington Day Hospital. It describes how a radical experiment in mental health democracy and liberty turned into anarchy, chaos and tyranny through the control of a manipulative and ultimately dangerous psychiatrist and analyst, 'Adrian' (Goodburn).[10] Baron argues that under his leadership, the staff operated implicit psychoanalytic rules which acted as a coercive regime of truth in the day hospital. The pursuit of these ideas ultimately led to a situation in which some patients felt neglected, mistreated and eventually led to an official enquiry and the eventual sacking of the medical director and the closure of the day hospital.

The term *asylum to anarchy* can be used, not only to refer to Baron's account of Paddington Day Hospital, but also more generally as a narrative that has been drawn upon to describe and analyse 'failed' radical initiatives, and most particularly the fall from grace of the radical innovator (Spandler, 2006). Such 'stories of radical failure' can also be referred to as trickster stories. Trickster stories have been described as moral tales of radical failure which reveal and re-affirm the very norms, belief systems and rules that are being broken and subverted (Hynes, 1993). In many ways, these stories actually serve as a model for the sanctity of the rules, because they vividly demonstrate what

---

9. It could be argued that some ideas from 'anti-psychiatry' have been effectively co-opted, thus reducing its more fundamental challenge to the legitimacy of psychiatric knowledge.
10. Goodburn has entered folklore through two trickster narratives. Not only through the dangerous psychoanalyst in *Asylum to Anarchy*, but also the charming but ultimately flawed 'Adrian Goodlove' in Erica Jong's *Fear of Flying* (Jong, 1974). In both narratives he signified the disappointment and false hopes represented by individual men and psychotherapy, however seemingly 'radical'.

happens if these rules are broken (Hynes & Doty, 1993). In these stories, the trickster figure ends up being banished from the community because he takes it upon himself to break the rules upon which the social order depends:

> Sooner or later the violator must pay a price for his violations ... Therefore, he must be depicted as falling into his own traps, the victim of his own ruses, and that can be expressed narratively only as being a result of silly and awkward comportment ... he appears as a being who lacks common sense, acting inconsistently and absurdly. (Makarius, 1993: 84)

Baron's *Asylum to Anarchy* is littered with many possible illustrations of this; for example, what appear to be far-fetched and mocking interpretations of patients' motives in the day hospital. Whilst convincingly argued, Baron's account can be criticised for being an ahistorical account which portrayed a one-sided view, both of the radical psychiatrist, who is portrayed predominantly as a destructive, infantile figure, and the day hospital itself, which is portrayed as a disastrous experiment in democracy. In particular, it did not take into account some of the positive developments and innovations that were initiated and supported at the day hospital, such as the development of the Mental Patients' Union (Spandler, 2006).

Moreover, her account has functioned as a trickster story because it seemed to demonstrate that attempts at subverting dominant (psychiatric) norms and values merely reinforces the necessity of these norms (Hynes & Doty, 1993). Thus such stories serve to maintain the status quo by making it appear self-evident and necessary. For many mental health workers, particularly those in the therapeutic community field, *Asylum to Anarchy* seemed to justify the need to bring greater conformism into practice. Specifically, it suggested that the challenges to psychiatric convention that the day hospital set in motion might be dangerous, and therefore practices of permissiveness and libertarianism should be curtailed, and greater structures and rules implemented (Spandler, 2006). Indeed, Baron herself argues that her analysis seemed to 'illustrate the ... irrationality of more democratic psychiatric methods' (Baron, 1984: 157). In addition, despite there being no serious consequences or catastrophes in the day hospital under Goodburn, *Asylum to Anarchy* operated as an 'atrocity story' which played into the hands of a growing conservatism in the 1980s which made innovation and experimentation more difficult.[11] It has been noted how 'atrocity stories' often function in society as a way to silence or close down spaces for debate and possible innovation in thinking (White & Featherstone, 2005; White, 2006).

Although I call this a 'trickster story of radical failure', I do not necessarily argue that it is completely 'untrue', nor that such radical practices actually 'succeeded' in any simplistic way. However, I do argue that these accounts overplay the element of failure at the expense of a genuine attempt at a serious and critical appraisal of radical innovations

---

11. Although another paradox of this period was that increasing consumerism helped pave the way for a stronger 'service user' movement in the 1980s (Campbell, 1996; Rogers & Pilgrim, 1991).

in and against mainstream psychiatry. It is too easy to either discard radical innovations into the dustbin of history of a more optimistic and radical past, or to romanticise such developments as a sense of nostalgia for things past.

Rather, it is important to try and develop accounts which re-inscribe the trickster with their essentially paradoxical qualities, both positive and negative, constructive and destructive. Indeed one of the ultimate paradoxes at the heart of the Paddington Day Hospital story was that it was a group of patients, those who the day hospital had sought to 'empower', who initiated a complaint into the functioning of the day hospital which eventually led to Goodburn being sacked and the day hospital closing down. Goodburn represented and re-created the aspirations and disappointments of radical psychiatry. Despite this, the radical psychiatrist as trickster has played an important role in challenging psychiatric thinking and practice. Whether this remains to be true is discussed in the next section.

CULTIVATING TRICKSTER SENSIBILITIES

Whilst it can be argued that figures such as Laing, Cooper and Szasz, as well as Goodburn, could be referred to as tricksters, it is harder to find examples of female psychiatrists who could be described in this way. It would, of course, be a bitter irony if the ultimate challenge to psychiatry was limited to white, male and middle-class psychiatrists. This is another paradox of the psychiatrist as trickster. More generally, as we have already noted, there is a lack of women tricksters in cultural mythologies and narratives, which might serve to limit its effectiveness as a concept with which to understand resistance and innovation. It would be too simplistic to assume that this lack refers to any 'essential' gender differences between men and women. It may be that the idea of the trickster is too narrow and misses its female expression (i.e. we need to look more widely to find them), or that when 'trickster energy' is manifested in a female body they are not viewed as tricksters. In part, this is because culturally and historically, women have been legally and socially excluded from particular roles in society and from our collective consciousness (Tannen, 2007). In other words, it is actually harder for women, not only to command such roles in societies that are riddled with gender inequalities, but even to be created in this role in our collective cultural imagination.

Therefore, one of the many limitations of the individual 'charismatic leader' or 'trickster' is that it touches on the old myth of the 'great man'. If, as Radin argues, 'every generation occupies itself with interpreting trickster anew' (Radin, cited in Hyde, 1998: 3), then we need to consider new expressions of tricksters in the modern context. For example, Sue White has argued that the reflexive social work practitioner can operate as a trickster in order to challenge the underlying assumptions and contradictions inherent in their profession. She argues that health and welfare work in general (and the case could be argued particularly strongly in psychiatric practice) is riddled with ambiguity and it needs trickster figures to ensure that these ambiguities are confronted:

> The important message about the trickster myths ... is that they are a celebration and a reminder of the need to open up dialogue and reflective spaces *within one's own culture*, to be anthropological about one's own suppositions. It is easy to spot the flaws in the practices of others, but the capacity of cultures to act as sustaining media for established forms of thought means that for us all, as members of cultures many of our own taken-for-granted distinctions never receive scrutiny. (White, 2006: 24)

Thus tricksters are necessary in order to open up (and keep open) reflexive spaces to challenge hegemonic practices, to 'spot a new orthodoxy and trouble its unintended consequences' (White, 2006: 30). Rather than seeing the trickster as an individual crusader we should look instead at the variety of ways in which it is possible to express trickster qualities within mental health practice. This requires us to consider the current spaces that are available for the expression of the creative and innovative energies which are necessary to challenge orthodoxies in theory and practice.

Ultimately this 'democratises' the notion of the trickster, seeing it as a position that might be available to different people at different times. Thus, rather than looking for new trickster *figures*, we might need to look at ways of engendering new trickster *sensibilities*. As White has argued, this is important in order to keep open important debates and paradoxes in professional practice, rather than prematurely close them off, or deny their existence. Whilst the idea of a truly *democratic* psychiatry (or society) might always be more aspiration than facticity, a 'trickster politics of tensions' keeps alive the question of democracy's *possibility*, by broadening and deepening spaces for durable radical democratic engagement in practice (Coles, 2006: 557–9). Cultivating a trickster sensibility would entail:

> [T]he ability to craft vision, practice, and power by sustaining a series of important tensions. This construction of democracy-in-tension promises a responsiveness, suppleness, and mobility that might just develop the power to help bring forth a better world. (Coles, 2006: 547)

CONCLUSION

On a number of different levels the notion of the trickster helps us to understand how we might confront the various tensions or troubled relations that are apparent in the struggle for more democratic mental health services. Ultimately it might help generate a greater understanding of the conditions of possibility for present and future sites of contestation, within and beyond psychiatric contexts. Cultivating a democratised 'trickster sensibility' might be one way of challenging current thinking and practices, keeping open our ability to question and not enforcing premature 'solutions' to our necessary and profound uncertainty in the field of mental health care.

REFERENCES

Alaszewski, A, Manthorpe, J & Walsh, M (1995) Risk: The sociological view of perception and management. *Nursing Times, 91*, 47.

Baron, C (1984) The Paddington Day Hospital: Crisis and control in a therapeutic institution. *International Journal of Therapeutic Communities, 5* (3), 157–70.

Baron, C (1987) *Asylum to Anarchy.* London: Free Association Books.

Brown, T & Hanvey, C (1987) The spirit of the times: Ten years after Case Con. *Community Care*, July, 18–19.

Burston, D (1996) *The Wing of Madness: The life and work of RD Laing.* Cambridge, MA/London: Harvard University Press.

Burstow, B (2005) Feminist antipsychiatry praxis: Women and the movement(s). In W Chan, D Chunn & R Menzies (Eds) *Women, Madness and the Law: A feminist reader* (pp 245–58). London: Glasshouse Press.

Campbell, P (1996) The history of the user movement in the United Kingdom. In T Heller, J Reynolds, R Gomm, R Muston & S Pattison (Eds) *Mental Health Matters* (pp 218–25). Basingstoke: Macmillan.

Coles, R (2006) Of tension and tricksters: Grassroots democracy between theory and practice. *Perspectives on Politics, 4* (3), 547–61.

Cooper, D (1967) *Psychiatry and Anti-Psychiatry.* London: Tavistock Publications.

Cooper, D (1978) *The Language of Madness.* London: Allen Lane, Penguin.

Cresswell, M (2008) Szasz and his interlocutors: Reconsidering Thomas Szasz's 'myth of mental illness' thesis. *Journal for the Theory of Social Behaviour, 38* (1), 23–44.

Crossley, N (1998) RD Laing and the British anti-psychiatry movement: A socio-historical analysis. *Social Science and Medicine, 47*, 877–99.

Crossley, N (1999) Fish, field, habitus and madness: The first wave mental health users movement. *British Journal of Sociology, 50* (4), 647–70.

Doty WG & Hynes WJ (1993) Historical overview of theoretical issues: The problem of the trickster. In WJ Hynes & WG Doty (Eds) *Mythical Trickster Figures: Contours, contexts and criticisms* (pp 13–32). Tuscaloosa, AL/London: University of Alabama Press.

Durkin, L (1972) Patient power: Review of a protest. *Social Work Today, 3* (15), 14.

Freeman, J (1984) The tyranny of structurelessness. In J Freeman & C Levine *Untying the Knot: Feminism, anarchism and organisation* (pp 5–16). London: Dark Star Press and Rebel Press. (Original work published 1974)

Freeman, J (1999) On the origins of social movements. In J Freeman & V Johnson (Eds) *Waves of Protest: Social movements since the sixties* (pp 7–24). Lanham, MD: Rowman and Littlefield.

Goffman, E (1961) *Asylums: Essays on the social situation of mental patients and other inmates.* Harmondsworth: Penguin.

Haddon, B (1979) Political implications of therapeutic communities. In RD Hinshelwood & N Manning (Eds) *Therapeutic Communities: Reflections and progress* (pp 1–15). London: Routledge and Kegan Paul.

Hinshelwood, RD (1987) *What Happens in Groups? Psychoanalysis, the individual and the community.* London: Free Association Books.

Hobson, RF (1979) The messianic community. In RD Hinshelwood & N Manning (Eds) *Therapeutic Communities: Reflections and progress* (pp 231–44). London: Routledge and Kegan Paul.

Hyde, L (1998) *Trickster Makes the World: Mischief, myth and art.* New York: North Point Press.
Hynes, WJ (1993) Mapping the characteristics of mythic tricksters: A heuristic guide. In WJ Hynes & WG Doty (Eds) *Mythical Trickster Figures: Contours, contexts and criticisms* (pp 33–45). Tuscaloosa, AL/London: University of Alabama Press.
Hynes, WJ & Doty, WG (Eds) (1993) *Mythical Trickster Figures: Contours, contexts and criticisms.* Tuscaloosa, AL/London: University of Alabama Press.
Jenner, FA, Moneiro, ACD, Zagalo-Cardosa, JA & Cunha-Oliveira, JA (1993) *Schizophrenia: A disease or some ways of being human?* Sheffield: Sheffield Academic Press.
Jong, E (1974) *Fear of Flying.* New York: Granada.
Jung, CG (1955) On the psychology of the trickster figure. In P Radin *The Trickster: A study in American Indian mythology* (pp 195–211). New York: Schocken.
Kennard, D (1991) The therapeutic community impulse: A recurring democratic tendency in troubled times. *Changes, 1,* 33–43.
Kopp, S (1976) The trickster-healer. In EWL Smith (Ed) *The Growing Edge of Gestalt Therapy* (pp 69–83). New York: Brunner/Mazel.
Leitner, M (1999) Pathologising as a way of dealing with conflicts and dissent in the psychoanalytic movement. *Free Associations, 7* (3), 459–83.
Lorde, A (2000) The master's tools will never dismantle the master's house. In K-K Bhavnani *Feminism and Race* (pp 89–92). Oxford: Oxford University Press.
Makarius, L (1993) The myth of the trickster: The necessary breaker of taboos. In WJ Hynes & WG Doty (Eds) *Mythical Trickster Figures: Contours, contexts and criticisms* (pp 66–86). Tuscaloosa, AL/London: University of Alabama Press.
Melucci, A (1994) A strange kind of newness: What's 'new' in new social movements? In E Laraña, H Johnston & JR Gusfield (Eds) *New Social Movements: From ideology to identity* (pp 101–30). Philadelphia, PA: Temple University Press.
Melucci, A (1996) *Challenging Codes: Collective action in the information age.* Cambridge: Cambridge University Press.
Mezan, P (1972) After Freud and Jung, now comes RD Laing. *Esquire, 77,* 92–178.
Miller, P & Rose, N (Eds) (1986) *The Power of Psychiatry.* London: Polity Press.
Mosher, LR (1991) In memoriam: RD Laing. An anti-psychiatrist's contribution to contemporary psychiatry. *International Journal of Therapeutic Communities, 12* (1), 43–51.
Mullan, B (Ed) (1997) *RD Laing: Creative destroyer.* London: Cassell.
Norton, K (1992) A culture of enquiry — Its preservation or loss. *Therapeutic Communities, 13,* 3–25.
Parker, I, Georgaca, E, Harper, D, McLaughlin, T & Stowell-Smith, M (1995) *Deconstructing Psychopathology.* London: Sage.
Radin, P (1955) *The Trickster: A study in American Indian mythology.* New York: Schocken.
Rogers, A & Pilgrim, D (1991) Pulling down churches: Accounting for the British mental health users' movement. *Sociology of Health and Illness, 13,* 29–48.
Rose, G (1993) *Feminism and Geography: The limits of geographical knowledge.* Minneapolis, MN: University of Minnesota Press.
Routledge, P (2003) Convergence space: Process geographies of grassroots globalization networks. *Transactions of the Institute of British Geographers, 28,* 333–49
Showalter, E (1987) *The Female Malady.* London: Virago.
Spandler, H (2001) Julian, not Adrian. Julian Goodburn: An appreciation. *Therapeutic Communities, 22* (4), 335–7.

Spandler, H (2002) Asylum to action: Paddington Day Hospital, therapeutic communities and beyond. PhD thesis, Department of Psychology and Speech Pathology, Manchester Metropolitan University.

Spandler, H (2006) *Asylum to Action: Paddington Day Hospital, therapeutic communities and beyond.* London/Philadelphia, PA: Jessica Kingsley.

Tannen, RS (2007) *The Female Trickster: The mask that reveals.* London/New York: Routledge.

Thomas, T (2002) Dead men laughing? Reflections of the praxis of Henry Ezriel and Julian Goodburn. *Therapeutic Communities, 23* (3), 219–24.

Warner, R (1994) *Recovery from Schizophrenia: Psychiatry and political economy.* London: Routledge.

White, S (2006) Unsettling reflections: The reflexive practitioner as 'trickster' in interprofessional work. In S White, J Fook & F Gardner (Eds) *Critical Reflection in Health and Social Care* (pp 21–39). Milton Keynes: Open University Press.

White, S & Featherstone, B (2005) Communicating misunderstandings: Multi-agency work as social work practice. *Child and Family Social Work, 10,* 207–16.

Zimberoff, D & Hartman, D (2003) Gestalt therapy and heart-centred therapies. *Journal of Heart-Centred Therapies, 6* (1), 93–104.

CHAPTER 7

WRITING FROM THE ASYLUM
A RE-ASSESSMENT OF THE VOICES OF FEMALE PATIENTS IN THE HISTORY OF PSYCHIATRY IN FRANCE

Susannah Wilson

In 1838 a law was passed in France that for the first time defined insanity in medico-legal terms. The law offered a legal conception of madness as a pathological state requiring treatment by medical professionals, and as a potential danger to society necessitating the incarceration of those afflicted. This law allowed for mandatory committal to public asylums upon the agreement of either two doctors and an agent of the law (the 'Official Committal'), or one family member and one doctor (the so-called 'Voluntary Committal') (Castel, 1976: 316–24).[1]

The early nineteenth century is a period traditionally viewed as one of great progress in the history of French psychiatry.[2] Clinicians were beginning to argue that dealing with insanity was not just an issue of policing and controlling, but that medical treatment offered hope to those who had previously been judged incurable. Practitioners such as Philippe Pinel believed that if mental illness could be understood, then it could be cured. The image of Pinel literally unshackling the insane has become a mythical notion that recurs in the historiography of French psychiatry.[3] There is little evidence that this legendary event actually took place, but the metaphorical image of the alienist doctor represents the ideal of liberation from the shackles of a disturbed mind through medical treatment.[4] This was indeed an ambitious aim, and there can be little doubt that the ideology of the asylum was founded on the Enlightenment ideal of progress in a healing, therapeutic space.

---

1. This chapter is in part based on work previously completed for a forthcoming monograph entitled *Voices from the Asylum: Four French Women Writers, 1850–1920*, and is reproduced with the kind permission of Oxford University Press.
2. This view of the history of psychiatry in France—that presents the advancement of knowledge in this field as fundamentally enlightened and progressive—is represented by critics such as Semelaigne, 1930–32.
3. Two famous paintings depict this scene. Charles Muller, *Pinel releases from their shackles the insane of Bicêtre*, is displayed at the Académie de Médecine, Paris. Robert Fleury, *Pinel delivering the insane*, is held by the Assistance Publique, Hôpitaux de Paris.
4. For a critical analysis of the formation of this myth, see Swain, 1997: 151–93 and Weiner, 1994. The term 'psychiatrist' was used in France as early as 1802, but limited to scholarly discourse, and did not come into common usage until 1900. The earliest use of the term 'psychiatry' was in 1847 (Goldstein, 1987: 6–7). The standard term used for asylum doctors was 'alienist'.

However, by the late nineteenth century criticism of the law of 1838 had become widespread. Causing particular alarm was the apparent ease with which it was possible to commit a person indefinitely to an asylum, and a significant debate in the French press ensued about the power of the police and the psychiatrist.[5] This public discussion echoed the voices of many patients who felt their detention was unwarranted, and lively written exchanges regarding the asylum ensued from within and without its walls (Fauvel, 2002).

In 1845, the distinguished alienist Moreau de Tours (1845: 133) seems to have asserted the importance of listening more to the patient's voice: 'If the insane have at times spoken, we have not taken sufficient account of what they have said.' It is perhaps ironic, from the point of view of the patient, that he should have made this recommendation: Murat (2001: 182) has shown that between the passing of the new law in 1838 and 1870, the number of women incarcerated in public asylums doubled; the decades of the 1860s and 1870s also saw a marked increase in the number of patients, male and female, writing in objection to their incarceration (Rigoli, 2001: 413). Few examples of writing by female patients have survived, and this paper will examine the cases of two women, Hersilie Rouy and Camille Claudel, who were subjected to long periods of incarceration and who wrote extensively in protest against their forced detention. Their narratives are complex utterances that offer simultaneously a compelling critique of the psychiatric treatment they received, and disturbing delusional accounts that reflect the suffering they endured at the hands of a society antagonistic to the aspirations of women. The 'delusional' nature of these accounts can be read as an act of symbolic resistance against a system of medical treatment that functioned as an integral part of a misogynistic society, and if not as literally true, then indeed as metaphorical expressions of lived experiences. These manifest themselves primarily as paranoid delusions of persecution (Claudel) and grandeur (Rouy), which may be read as metaphorical representations of real abuse, or as compensatory devices constructed to ensure the survival of the self against the threat of social or mental annihilation.

The patients' narratives examined here were also produced in the context of the enduring legacy of the Napoleonic Civil Code, established from 1800 to 1804, which was in many ways regressive, relegating women to the status of a minor. The code stated that a woman owed her husband obedience in exchange for his protection. Although it had previously been legal, divorce was made illegal and remained so until 1884; in addition, women could not legally pursue the estranged father of a child (Zeldin, 1973: 343–62). The problem of marriage and illegitimacy was exacerbated, of course, by the illegality of abortion and the non-existence of reliable contraception.

The cases presented here are women whose stories have a number of important common points: both transgressed the gender stereotypes laid down by patriarchal society by failing in their functions as 'normal' bourgeois women. They were unmarried and

---

5. The case of Hersilie Rouy received particular attention in the press. *France Médicale* (12 August 1871: 369–73) published a piece defending the health professionals involved in her case, and a response from Rouy was also printed. *Le Figaro* also published a story sympathetic to Rouy's ordeal on 28 July 1871. Sérieux and Capgras (1910: 221) lament the press involvement in her case: 'The local newspapers tell of the odious persecutions endured by this victim ... she has become the heroine of the day.'

childless, although both engaged in extra-marital affairs and, as we shall later examine, there is significant anecdotal evidence to suggest that they both fell pregnant at some stage: Sérieux and Capgras (1910: 195–96) say in their case history that Rouy is likely to have lost a child; and Claudel's brother alludes to her having had at least one abortion (Antoine, 1988: 166). They were interested in art, culture and learning and in reaching beyond the constraints of the private sphere. These case studies show that each of these authors was alienated within society, having failed to meet the requirements of culturally constructed feminine normality, before being alienated from herself through serious mental illness.

HERSILIE ROUY

The case of Hersilie Rouy (1814–1881) is discussed at some length in treatises by the most famous clinicians of the time, particularly in contemporary debates on the incipient concept of paranoia. She exhibited some evidence of delusions of grandeur, specifically the belief that she was the changeling child of French aristocrats. This recreating of one's family history was famously theorised by Freud as a 'family romance' scenario, 'which finds expression in a phantasy in which both his parents are replaced by others of better birth. The technique used in developing phantasies like this ... depends upon the ingenuity and the material which the child has at his disposal' (Freud, 1909: 239). She was also mentioned in discussions of afflictions labelled 'lucid madness' (Trélat, 1861: 183–6), 'behavioural madness', and 'reasoning madness' (Sérieux & Capgras, 1909: 386).

Rouy wrote a five-hundred-page account of her time spent in various psychiatric institutions in Paris and the French provinces between 1854 and 1868, entitled *Memoirs of a Madwoman* (Rouy, 1883). The book was published some years after her death, and the title conferred by her editor is ironic given that she vociferously denied she was insane, and from the moment of her incarceration until the day she died fought for her sanity to be recognised and to pursue in law those she considered to be responsible for her committal. Rouy was a talented musician who was working as a piano teacher in 1854, when upon her father's death her family discovered that she and her sister were illegitimate, thus negating the will and their inheritance. After a period of conflict with her half-brother and sister, Rouy claims that she was unexpectedly taken away by a doctor and admitted to the private asylum at Charenton under her mother's maiden name of 'Chevalier'. She was soon transferred to the Salpêtrière, the women's public asylum in Paris, as an 'official committal'. Whilst incarcerated, the doctors treating her despaired of her rebellious behaviour and seemingly obsessive letter writing, and were wearied by her intransigence in protest against their authority. Rouy managed to secure her release for two reasons: first, she managed to gain allies through her relentless letter writing, most notably Edouard Le Normant des Varannes, who held an important administrative position at the Orléans asylum, and who would later publish her memoirs; second, the medical professionals dealing with her seem to have given up on her treatment, preferring to release her deemed 'cured', despite the fact that they unanimously considered her to be still psychiatrically ill.

After her release, Rouy dedicated the remainder of her life to writing up her memoirs for publication and fighting for compensation, which eventually she won. She died in 1881 and was buried with her father's name, which she fought hard to retain, and with the recognition that she was his legitimate daughter.[6] Unlike most of her female contemporaries in the asylum, Rouy was vindicated: 'cured', released, and compensated for her troubles. Rouy may be viewed either as an insane, insubordinate troublemaker, or as a sane person falsely committed to the asylum without good reason. Arguably, however, engaging with the delusional aspect of her story reveals as much about the injustice of her suffering as do the more straightforward details of her case.

A detailed examination of Rouy's case history reveals that events prior to her committal certainly seem to have precipitated a 'breakdown': she lost her mother at a formative age; just before her committal she lost a father to whom she was especially close; she discovered that her parents had not been legally married; losing her inheritance which plunged her into financial insecurity, she lived a precarious life with an unreliable income; she had a relationship with a man who left her when she was pregnant, and the baby died soon after it was born. At the age of 34, having lost everything that meant anything real to her, Rouy locked herself away in her home and began to construct a whole new life story for herself based on the delusional interpretation of her birth and baptism certificates. A neighbour alerted the police; they forced entry into her apartment and found her kneeling in front of a little coffin shrouded in black, surrounded by lighted candles. She was examined by a doctor and taken to the private asylum at Charenton (Sérieux & Capgras, 1910: 193–225).

Rouy's case is, in some respects, a classic case of paranoia where the patient's sanity appeared sufficiently plausible to convince many on the outside that she was being falsely detained. However, she also developed a delusional narrative, to which she refers extensively but also claims paradoxically not to believe. It seems that Rouy came to imagine that she was the lost daughter of the Duchess of Berry, mother of the pretender to the Bourbon throne. In 1820 (six years after Rouy's birth), the Duke of Berry had been murdered during his wife's pregnancy, and rumours had circulated at the time of the birth of the Duchess's son that a child swap had been carried out to ensure a male heir (Merriman, 1985: 53–7).

Rouy's account reveals the double bind in which patients found themselves vis-à-vis the clinical observer: her claim to be sane, and the dissimulation of her delusional ideas, are taken as symptomatic of her mental illness. There is no linguistic space in which she can express the truth of her experience and be believed. In a letter addressed to the popular Empress and wife of Napoleon III, Eugénie, and reproduced in her memoirs, Rouy thematises the circumstances of her birth, the beginning of her life and her precarious sense of identity. Her writing expresses a paradoxical anxiety, that of appearance in the world and disappearance, the concern of belonging and the terror of being eradicated:

---

6. Rouy's father seems to have married her mother without having divorced his first wife, making his subsequent children technically illegitimate. Rouy was officially recognised as legitimate at the end of her life, ironically perhaps, on her death certificate. This is noted by the editor of her memoirs (Rouy, 1883: 491).

> After the assassination of the Duke of Berry, the duchess, his wife, gave birth to a son and a daughter. It is not necessary, Madam, to remind you of the position of the Royal Family at the moment, in order for you to understand the absolute necessity of sacrificing the poor daughter for the good of France. She was therefore kidnapped from the King's Palace and hidden from view. However, a child was seen *being taken away*, and because the secret was not kept, rumours of a child swap took the place of the sad truth. (Rouy, 1883: 168)[7]

Rouy goes on to explain how this child ended up being taken away to Russia and adopted by the Rouy family (who lived in Russia during Hersilie's early childhood), where she grew up happily. She frequently notes that this child was seen to be special or gifted, perhaps different in some way: 'As the child was growing up, Madam, her striking resemblance with the Duchess of Berry surprised everybody, and this reminded them of the malicious rumours that had circulated around the time of her birth' (Rouy, 1883: 169). Rouy is careful to distance herself from the idea of a child substitution, and projects the process of deduction onto people around her; she makes frequent reference to her own physical appearance, and to features that made her stand out as a child: her 'curly blonde hair' and her nickname, 'Golden Star' (Rouy, 1883: 32). These seemingly narcissistic references contrast strongly with the fate that Rouy claims would befall the abducted child, whose existence was always threatened:

> And when the astronomer [Rouy's father], sole protector of the young abandoned woman, died, no one dared to ask the woman who had unwittingly become a member of that family to abandon the name she had received from *the man* who had raised her tenderly, and someone kidnapped her; she was made to disappear and placed in one of those prisons that have outlived the Old Regime; someone locked her away in a mental asylum, under the name of *Chevalier, of unknown parents*. (Rouy, 1883: 169)

Rouy's delusions serve as a form of metaphorical compensation for what she had suffered at the hands of a family that abandoned her, and a society in which her musical ambition had no real outlet. Her stories of child substitution translate into the idea, 'my existence is legitimate', and her inflated sense of her status in the world functions as a metaphorical reversal of the experience of social annihilation.

The experience of being committed to the asylum under what Rouy considered to be a false name, *Chevalier*, and of being declared of unknown parentage, seems to have been a particularly shattering experience. The dissolution of her sense of identity becomes clear later in the text of her memoirs, where she testifies to having adopted different names and corresponding identities in order to draw attention to her case. In addition to the aforementioned childhood nickname of 'Golden Star', which recurs throughout the text, Rouy at different points in her story signs her letters with a bizarre range of

---

7. All emphases are the author's own. Translations from the original French texts are mine.

names, including some borrowed from the Italian *Commedia dell'arte*: 'Punchinello', 'Satan', 'The Antichrist', 'The Sylphid', 'The Siren', 'The Saltimbanco' (acrobat), and 'Sister of King Henry V' (Rouy, 1883: 264–5). The partial adoption (for Rouy claims never to really believe she is any of these people) of these multiple identities seems to lend power to the weakened self, and to disrupt the administrative procedure of the asylum that has named her 'Chevalier'.

These characters exercise power over those around them, whether supernatural spiritual potency (Satan and the Antichrist) or the ultimate political power of the royal family. To parallel her own experience to that of the French royal family at this time in history is to draw an unconscious comparison between the precariousness of an institution under mortal threat with the insult done to her own sense of self. The remaining characters she assumes are manipulators and tricksters: the seductive siren; the evasive and flitting sylphid; the playful Punchinello and the acrobat. These traits reflect the strategies deployed by Rouy, whose use of multiple signatures and identities forms a counter-tactic aimed at outmanoeuvring the system that has named her 'Hersilie Chevalier-Rouy'; it is also subversive of the clinician's signature given on official statements. However, the multiple selves textually expressed are also indicative of the disintegration of the coherent sense of self that the process of attempted reparation called 'megalomania' produces. This results in the creation of a new 'me', constructed to mitigate the unbearable suffering of the real 'me'.[8]

Despite periodically returning to delusional ideas, in her memoirs Rouy also offers her reader a coherent critique of the reasoning processes motivating the decisions made by her doctors. In straightforward and precise terms, she damns their vague assessments of her state of mind. At the time of her admission to the Salpêtrière, Rouy tried to explain to those responsible that she had been admitted under the wrong name.[9] She was repeatedly ignored, and makes the key observation: 'Unfortunately, there as at Charenton, nobody takes any notice of what the inmates say' (Rouy, 1883: 98).

The initial committal certificate, signed by the distinguished alienist Ulysse Trélat, notes simply: 'Is affected by partial delirium'. This, as Rouy correctly points out, is simply copied from another statement made by the doctor who had assessed her at Charenton, Louis-Florentin Calmeil. This doctor gives us a little more detail, noting that Rouy is capable of holding a 'semi-coherent conversation', but that the rest of the time she is 'prey to the most erroneous ideas, and to the most unreasonable notions'; she also 'gives herself over to the most extravagant actions'. Calmeil considers it dangerous to leave her in the grip of her madness, and decides that her continued detention is necessary. As we have seen, there may well have been some truth in this assessment of

---

8. The psychoanalytical notion that 'megalomania' is the indirect result of emotional disappointment is outlined in Freud's 'Case History of Schreber' (1911: 65). Jung (1907: 145) puts forward an argument that resonates more closely with my own. In his 1907 analysis of the word associations of his patient Babette Staub, he observes that delusions of grandeur are compensatory: 'The conscious psychic activity of the patient, then, is limited to a systematic creation of wish-fulfilments as a substitute, so to speak, for a life of toil and privation and for the depressing experiences of a wretched family milieu.'
9. In fact, the documentation included at the end of the memoirs does confirm that 'Chevalier' is the maiden name of Rouy's mother, suggesting that, having been declared illegitimate, she had been given her mother's name without her own consent (Rouy, 1883: 494).

Rouy's state of mind. However, their condemnation leaves Rouy feeling abandoned and betrayed by those expected to defend her interests:

> He [Lasègue] only saw me for a minute or two, and only told me what I have just reported. He condemns me on the word of Doctor Calmeil, who condemns me on the word of a doctor, who, never having seen me, was kind enough to kidnap me at the request of someone else!

The overwhelming sense communicated in Rouy's account is that of never being taken seriously by clinicians. The certificate to legally commit Rouy (and reproduced in her memoirs) is a pro-forma document in which the blanks are filled with her name and personal details. The medical assessment is generic, and reads: '[Hersilie-Camille-Joséphine Chevalier-Rouy] is in a state of mental alienation that compromises public order or the safety of others, as noted in a statement by the police chief superintendent.' Rouy points out that there is nothing on the certificate that explicitly refers to her case, and notes the lack of specificity and personal engagement in the evaluation of her distress: 'The medical assessment is therefore the same for everyone.'[10]

Even at the end of her time in the asylum, after fighting for years to clear her name and gain her liberty, Rouy was released not because she was really thought to have recovered. She was considered incurable and the doctors, quite simply, wanted rid of her—perhaps because they could not envisage her being able to respond to any treatment they could offer her. Doctor Payen at the Orléans asylum describes her in the most unfavourable terms as:

> [A]n untreatable resident, and of the worst variety, because of the trouble she's always causing and because of the irrepressible insubordination that she exhibits. When this manifests itself in a person like this, who is as intelligent as she is persistent and determined, it is displayed in an attitude of arrogance, vanity and envy. All my colleagues and I consider this to be a type of incurable madness that ought to be contained within a mental asylum, and we would be very pleased if it were not the Orléans asylum. (Rouy, 1883: 443)

Of a list of personality traits that reads like an inventory of feminine vices, Rouy, perhaps proud of her status as arch-troublemaker, simply asks: 'where is the madness in that?' (Rouy, 1883: 443). The attitude of hostility and disbelief with which Rouy's ideas were repeatedly greeted actually seems to have exacerbated her problems, and made her delusions all the more entrenched, making the experience of 'asylum' that of existing in a pathogenic, rather than a therapeutic, space.

---

10. These medical records are all reproduced word-for-word in her memoirs (Rouy, 1883: 92–9).

CAMILLE CLAUDEL

Camille Claudel (1864–1943) was a gifted sculptor whose life was overshadowed by two significantly more famous men: her brother, the French poet Paul Claudel, and her teacher and lover, the sculptor Auguste Rodin. Her artistic activity in the public eye lasted from about 1882 to 1905. She had broken off relations with Rodin in 1899, and was attempting to establish an independent reputation and to distance herself from his artistic control. Her work was inevitably compared to that of Rodin, and his influence, that had once been productive and inspirational, eventually proved utterly destructive. She became progressively more isolated, and delusional, eventually neglecting her own physical well-being and locking herself away in her Paris home after the death of her devoted father in 1913. It was an agonising decision for her brother, as head of the family, to commit her to a private asylum outside Paris as a 'voluntary' committal later in the same year. She was diagnosed as suffering from 'paranoid psychosis', and the diagnosis remained unchanged until her death in 1943 in the asylum of Montdevergues in the south of France, where she had been transferred during the First World War and where she remained for the rest of her life. She never worked again, and her correspondence was only published in recent years (Rivière & Gaudichon, 2003).

Over the past three decades, the importance of her work has been recognised and celebrated in France, but this recognition has come too late for Claudel ever to know.[11] Her recurrent idea, which persisted long after Rodin's death and until she died, thirty years after being committed to the asylum, was that Rodin was persecuting her. The particular theme that recurs in her writing is that her artwork had been stolen, destroyed or unacknowledged: either physically taken from her studio or maliciously copied by other artists. The theme of her accusations betrays a strong sense of violation, almost violence, and injustice, as well as paranoia:

> Another year, I used to pay a kid to bring me wood; he saw a sketch that I was doing (*Woman with a Doe*). Every Sunday he went to Meudon to tell Mr Rodin all about what he'd seen. The result—none other than that year he had three life-sized versions of *Woman with a Doe*, textually modelled on my version, which earned him 100,000 francs. Another time, a cleaning lady drugged my coffee and made me sleep for twelve hours straight. During this time, the woman broke into my bathroom and took the *Woman at the Cross*. The result was three *Woman at the Cross* figures earning 100,000 francs. (Rivière, 2003: 242)[12]

---

11. Before Rivière published Claudel's correspondence in 2003, critics such as Delbée (1982), Paris (1984) and Cassar (1987) had started the process of rediscovering the importance of her life and work. The success of Nuytten's 1989 film *Camille Claudel* helped to make the artist a household name in France.
12. These extracts appear in an undated letter. Rivière, the editor of Claudel's correspondence, dates the letter around 1909. Even after Rodin's death in 1917, his persecution of Claudel remains a central theme in her writings.

There is no evidence that Rodin actually copied these works from Claudel, but the argument that she was cheated by him, as a part of a broader set of circumstances meaning that she could not fulfil her true potential, does hold some water. These ideas can be read as a metaphorical representation of what was stolen from her, by Rodin, her family, and by the failure of society to allow her a space in which she could be taken seriously as an artist. Art historical research has proven that to this day there are artworks attributed to Rodin that were actually produced by Claudel, but she has enjoyed little acknowledged influence on his work.[13] Her delusions of persecution seem to be one means of asserting the idea, 'I am important enough to persecute', in compensation for the lack of artistic recognition she received in her lifetime. Claudel's assured sense of the significance of her artwork has ironically been given credibility in recent years, where in France there has been a veritable resurrection of interest in her life and work.

Like Rouy, Claudel also offers the modern reader a compelling account of how it feels to be the subject of psychiatric diagnosis, particularly where this assessment is enmeshed with a set of value judgements about the lifestyle choices of women who sought independence and artistic recognition. The only part of her medical records to contain any detailed assessment of her mental state is the initial committal certificate. For the rest of her life, her records consist of nothing more than an annual recording of the enduring state of 'paranoid psychosis'. In the first instance, her committal was motivated by concerns about the deterioration of her physical health and personal hygiene, exacerbated by an increasingly isolated lifestyle. As Dr Michaux recorded on 7 March 1913:

> I ... certify that Mademoiselle Camille Claudel is suffering from an attack of serious intellectual disturbance; that she wears shabby clothes; that she is absolutely filthy, and certainly never washes; that she has sold all her furniture, apart from a sofa and a bed; ... that she spends her life completely locked away in her airless lodgings, where the shutters remain hermetically closed; that for several months now she has not gone out during the day, but occasionally goes out in the middle of the night; according to letters recently sent to her brother, and according to comments made by her concierge, she still feels terrorized by 'Rodin's gang'; that on several occasions over the past seven or eight years I have noted during my home visits that she believes herself to be persecuted; and that her state, that already places her in danger because of her lack of personal care and even basic sustenance, is now becoming dangerous for her neighbours, and that it will be necessary to commit her to an asylum. (Paris, 1984)[14]

---

13. Paris gives four examples of important works sculpted by Claudel and exhibited, even to this day, under Rodin's signature (Paris & de la Chapelle, 1990: 34). The critic Morhardt (cited in Bouté, 1995: 24–5) also suggests that Claudel contributed significantly to the final production of Rodin's masterpiece, 'The Gates of Hell'.

14. Claudel's medical records are reproduced in Reine Marie Paris (1984: 193–208). From 1913 to 1942 they record no change in her mental state. In 1943, a decline is noted prior to her death.

After her committal, Claudel never saw her mother or sister again, and received only intermittent visits from her brother, Paul. She corresponded regularly with him, and in her letters regularly begs to be allowed to come home to her family. Instead, she stayed in the asylum for the remaining thirty years of her life. Although she does seem to reveal some awareness of her mental suffering, by, for example, admitting that she could no longer work because of her madness, she also offers a painfully clear insight into the last years of her life. To Paul, she writes: 'Of the dream that was my life, this is the nightmare' (Rivière & Gaudichon, 2003: 307). She also rejects the assessment of her mental health based on negative value judgements about her lifestyle:

> I am reproached (oh what a terrible crime) for having lived alone, for having spent my life with cats, for having delusions of persecution! It's on the basis of these accusations that I have been incarcerated for five and a half years like a criminal, deprived of freedom, deprived of food, of warmth and of the most basic commodities. (Rivière, 2003: 278)

Although Claudel's committal was motivated by genuine concern, what she communicates in her letters is that, imperfect though her lifestyle and state of mind may have been, the asylum has curtailed her freedom and left her without a vital creative space. The asylum is not experienced as a therapeutic environment, but rather as a cruel punishment. This, understandably, is in turn experienced as a betrayal by those who are meant to protect her.

Despite their sufferings and failings, through their writing these women have gained important personal victories over the injustices of their era, even if this recognition has come too late. For Rouy and Claudel, psychiatric medicine functioned as a medico-legal arm of a society that oppressed women, particularly those who deviated from the narrow path of normality dictated by society. The construction of delusional stories can be read as an understandable and indeed 'appropriate' response, a compensatory defence adopted in reaction to a social situation that annihilated an individual's aspirations.

These partially delusional accounts are not meaningless or unconnected to the case histories of these patients. Instead of medical practitioners using patient's narratives to a diagnostic end, they could have been used as an indication of what the individual had suffered as a means to a therapeutic end. Rather, these women became increasingly sick, arguably as a result, in part, of the failure of medical professionals to place any value on what they had to say. Their delusions became and remained entrenched, suggesting that their false realities continued to serve the function of bolstering a fragile and unsupported sense of self. In this sense, psychiatry colluded with rather than worked against the limitations placed upon these women by French society at this time.

REFERENCES

Antoine, G (1988) *Paul Claudel ou l'Enfer du Génie*. Paris: Robert Laffont.
Bouté, G (1995) *Camille Claudel: Le miroir et la nuit*. Paris: Éditions de l'amateur–Éditions des catalogues raisonnés.
Cassar, J (1987) *Dossier Camille Claudel*. Paris: Librairie Séguier/Archimbaud.
Castel, R (1976) *L'Ordre Psychiatrique: L'âge d'or de l'aliénisme*. Paris: Les éditions de minuit.
Delbée, A (1982) *Une Femme*. Paris: Presses de la Renaissance.
Fauvel, A (2002) Le crime de Clermont et la remise en cause des asiles en 1880. *Revue d'Histoire Moderne et Contemporaine, 49*, 195–216.
Freud, S (1909) Family Romances. In J Strachey et al (Eds) *The Standard Edition of the Complete Psychological Works of Sigmund Freud, Vol 9* (pp 235–41). London: Vintage.
Freud, S (1911) The case history of Schreber. In J Strachey et al (Eds) *The Standard Edition of the Complete Psychological Works of Sigmund Freud, Vol 12* (pp 3–82). London: Vintage.
Goldstein, J (1987) *Console and Classify: The French psychiatric profession in the nineteenth century*. Cambridge: Cambridge University Press.
Jung, CG (1907) The psychology of dementia praecox. In RFC Hall, (Trans) *The Psychogenesis of Mental Disease* (pp 1–151). *The Collected Works of CG Jung, Vol 3*. London: Routledge.
Merriman, JM (1985) The miracle baby. In JM Merriman (Ed) *For Want of a Horse: Chance and humor in history* (pp 53–7). Lexington, MA: The Stephen Greene Press.
Moreau de Tours, J-J (1845) *Du Hachisch et de l'Aliénation Mentale. Études psychologiques*. Paris: Masson.
Murat, L (2001) *La Maison du Docteur Blanche*. Paris: Lattès.
Nuytten, B (Dir) (1989) *Camille Claudel*. Paris: Christian Fechner Films.
Paris, R-M (1984) *Camille Claudel*. Paris: Gallimard.
Paris, R-M & de la Chapelle, A (1990) *L'Œuvre de Camille Claudel, catalogue raisonné*. Paris: Éditions d'art et d'histoire Arhis/Éditions Adam Biro.
Rigoli, J (2001) *Lire le Délire*. Geneva: Arthème Fayard.
Rivière, A & Gaudichon, B (Eds) (2003) *Camille Claudel: Correspondance*. Paris: Gallimard.
Rouy, H (1883) *Mémoires d'une Aliénée*. Paris: Ollendorff.
Semelaigne, R (1930–32) *Les Pionniers de la Psychiatrie Française Avant et Après Pinel*. Paris: Baillière.
Sérieux, P & Capgras, J (1909) *Les Folies Raisonnantes: Le délire d'interprétation*. Paris: Alcan.
Sérieux, P & Capgras, J (1910) Roman et vie d'une fausse princesse. *Journal de Psychologie Normale et Pathologique, 7*, 193–225.
Swain, G (1997) *Le Sujet de la Folie: Naissance de la psychiatrie*. Paris: Calmann-Lévy.
Trélat, U (1861) *La Folie Lucide Étudiée et Considérée au Point de Vue de la Famille et de la Société*. Paris: Delahaye.
Weiner, DB (1994) 'Le geste de Pinel': The history of a psychiatric myth. In R Porter & MS Micale (Eds) *Discovering the History of Psychiatry* (pp 232–47). Oxford: Oxford University Press.
Zeldin, T (1973) *France 1848–1945: Volume One: Ambition, love and politics*. Oxford: Clarendon.

Chapter 8

MIRRORS OF SHAME
THE ACT OF SHAMING AND THE SPECTACLE OF FEMALE SEXUAL SHAME

Jocelyn Catty

'For day', quoth she 'night's scapes doth open lay;
And my true eyes have never practis'd how
To cloak offences with a cunning brow.

'They think not but that every eye can see
The same disgrace which they themselves behold;
And therefore would they still in darkness be,
To have their unseen sin remain untold;
For they their guilt with weeping will unfold,
And grave, like water that doth eat in steel,
Upon my cheeks what helpless shame I feel.'
(Shakespeare, *The Rape of Lucrece*, 1594/1960: ll. 750–6)

Lucrece's lament over her rape exemplifies the tortured relationship between shame and guilt and attests both to the need for shame to seek a hiding place and to the sense in which it is inexorably experienced as publicised or viewed. While Lucrece's belief in her guilt, disgrace and 'helpless shame' could be interpreted in the early twenty-first century as a common response to sexual trauma, in which the victim blames herself for her violation, it also finds an immediate context in the taste for women's sexual shame evidenced by poetry of the 1590s and a more general one in the development of ideas about women's identify and volition in the early modern period.

Psychological and psychoanalytic accounts of shame attend to it as an affect or focus on shame-proneness as a pathology; less attention is paid in such accounts to acts of shaming. I shall argue that the act of shaming highlights the interplay between exposure and concealment involved in shame and that this is highlighted by the association between shame and rape: perhaps the quintessential act of shaming. Finally, I shall argue that the act of shaming is an intrinsic feature of representations of shame. This, along with the shame inherent in the act of self-disclosure, has profound implications for clinical practice in mental health. I shall illustrate these arguments by focusing on the Elizabethan 'female complaint' poem: a genre which frequently plays with this insidious way in which representation itself imposes shame and of which female sexual shame is an explicit theme.

My focus on the female complaint, which foregrounds sexual shame by engaging with conflicting definitions of rape and female sexual identity, affords an opportunity to consider both the particular significance of shame for women, in its social and cultural context, and the act of shaming as distinct from the state of shame. In bringing the portrayal of women's sexual shame by Elizabethan male poets into conjunction with psychological and psychoanalytic perspectives, I shall not be seeking to use psychoanalytic theory as a means of interpreting the putative feelings of the poems' female characters. I shall instead be using psychoanalytic insights as a framework for looking at some of the origins of our ideas about shame in the early modern period, in order in turn to explore the implications of the latter for our current understanding of shame. I shall argue that the poems illustrate the way in which representing shame—particularly in a cultural context which emphasises spectacle and thus reinforces shame—is always potentially a re-shaming.

While authors in the 1590s deploy shame as part of an increasing preoccupation with identity, the male poets of the 'female complaint' genre create female characters to embody a particularly sexual shame and perpetuate a voyeuristic taste for such a condition. Rather than suggesting any seamless continuity between late sixteenth-century culture and our own, I suggest that these texts which so explicitly deal in shame may demonstrate the importance of the act of shaming, the bodily nature of shame and the shame inherent in the act of 'complaining'.

SHAME AND IDENTITY

While the root of the word 'shame' means 'to cover oneself' (Wurmser, 1981: 29), the range of definitions of the word exhibits a profound tension. 'Shame' may be defined as 'the painful emotion arising from the consciousness of something dishonouring' or as 'fear of offence against propriety', the latter relating to the archaic 'shamefastness' (modesty) (*OED*, 1989). It may alternatively be defined as 'disgrace, ignominy', including 'violation of a woman's honour' (ibid). It thus indicates the affects attendant upon a certain kind of disgrace, the fear of being disgraced and the disgrace itself, while the verb 'to shame' may mean 'to make ashamed' or 'to inflict or bring disgrace upon'.

The fundamental distinction between shame and guilt has been understood to rest on the role of the self, with the self being central to shame, whereas in guilt, the action done or not done is paramount (HB Lewis, 1971). Shame is seen as involving an internalised other, before whom we are shamed. In this way, we become an object during the experience of shame. Michael Lewis understands shame as the 'closure of the self-object circle', whereby we become 'the object as well as the subject of shame' (1992: 34).

Recent empirical literature has confirmed this distinction between shame and guilt. Shame has been understood as involving the mechanism of splitting, whereby the shameful person experiences him- or herself as all bad, whereas in guilt both good and bad can be conceived of as held within the same person; a healthy split between the person and their action then enables them to take reparative action, typical of depressive position functioning. Someone shamed thus 'seeks to hide the self from others' in an 'escapist response', while 'guilt is more likely to keep people constructively engaged in the interpersonal situation in hand' through the urge to make reparation (Tangney, 1995: 119–20). Shame and guilt are thus also both 'social' emotions, in the sense of 'self-concerning, partly physical responses, that are at the same time aspects of a moral or ideological attitude' (Levy & Rosaldo, 1983, cited in Pines, 1995: 348) and used to control human conduct as 'the most powerful ... regulators and boundary markers' (Pines, 1995: 347).

As Freud's description of shame as 'considered to be a feminine characteristic *par excellence* but ... far more a matter of convention' (1933/1964: 132) may have anticipated, psychological accounts of shame which lack a sociological understanding of women's place in culture may be insufficient to understand the association between women and shame to which modern empirical research as well as much early modern literature attests. Sandra Lee Bartky has argued that psychologists have failed to treat shame 'in its relationship to oppression' (Bartky, 1990: 97). Not only are women more characterised by both shame and guilt than men, but 'some of the commoner forms of shame in men ... may be intelligible only in light of the presupposition of male power, while in women shame may well be a mark and token of powerlessness' (ibid: 84). The act of shaming may thus be effected culturally as well as by individuals.

Bartky argues that, for women, shame is a 'profound mode of disclosure both of self and situation' (ibid: 85). Disclosure, or uncovering, is central to the experience of shame, which involves a contradictory dynamic between hiding and exposure, covering and display. Leon Wurmser argues that shame 'guards the boundary of privacy' but also that it 'may pertain to the activity of exposing oneself' (1981: 59). This argument is in a sense a return to Freud's original view of shame as a reaction formation against exhibitionism (Freud, 1905/1953: 162). If shame intrinsically involves exposure, then it is always in a sense made visible or embodied; and embodiment is a particular focus for shame, especially for women. Women, Bartky argues, are vulnerable to 'the peculiar dialectic of shame and pride in embodiment consequent upon a narcissistic assumption of the body as spectacle' (1990: 84). This is nowhere more evident than in the phenomenon of body dysmorphic disorder (BDD) or bodily shame, a uniquely embodied form of pathological shame in which the sufferer becomes fixated on hated features of their body. Rozsika Parker has argued that BDD finds a context in contemporary Western culture's provision of 'a matrix within which the disorder can flourish' (2003: 452) through its emphasis on the spectacle of the female body. Embodiment is, conversely, a particular feature of shame in both genders, its salient features being blushing and averting the gaze: physiology and affect, internal and external deeply interrelated.

Acts of shaming in most of these accounts receive less attention than the internal state of shame. The high association of shame with rape and abuse, however, may challenge or extend these definitions. Phil Mollon argues that 'sexual abuse is the ultimate shame' and that its purpose may thus be 'to transfer projectively shame from the abuser to the victim' (1996: 54). Paul Gilbert also argues that abuse 'can be experienced like an (inner) disfigurement' (2002: 32). Conversely, a sense of violation seems to be central to the experience of shame as an affect, Mollon describing 'violation of the core self' (2002: 7) being experienced as rape, while Pines argues that a shameful thought is a violation of one's ideals: 'shame protects our own integrity and tells us if we have been invaded and exploited as well as telling us that we have failed to earn our self-respect' (1995: 350).

Malcolm Pines points out that 'the re-emergence of shame in our [psychoanalytic] literature accompanies the attention now given to identity and the self' (1995: 351). This interconnection between shame and identity is so strong that Ewan Fernie argues that in literature, shame's 'power fluctuates through time with the premium put on selfhood' (2002: 8). This may account for the emergence of shame as a major literary theme in the early modern period: a period which witnessed a rapid development of conceptions of selfhood (not just identity, but the degree to which that identity could be conceptualised as a sense of coherent self). The idea of shame in the early modern period, Fernie argues, gains added power from the fact that it was an age of display and spectacle: 'the early modern subject ... is very much constructed in the eyes of others' (2002: 57).

The tension between public shame (in the eyes of the world) and private shame (in one's own eyes) is played out in the female complaint, which displays a self-conscious awareness of the implications of spectacle. Whether a woman is the subject or the object of a poem in which she is held up as a figure of shame will prove to be an issue with which the poems themselves engage.

THE FEMALE COMPLAINT AND SEXUAL SHAME

The female complaint or lament is characterised by a preoccupation with female sexual shame and distress. The poems simultaneously celebrate and condemn female sexual misfortune, be it seduction or rape. This preoccupation finds a context in the sexualisation of literature in the Elizabethan period, particularly the 1590s, when texts 'self-consciously deal in the shameful ... [and] draw attention to their shamefulness' as a 'strategy of authorial self-promotion' (Brown, 2004: 2). Shame is associated with anxiety about exposure through publication in this, the age in which the printed text proliferated (Wall, 1993).

The complaint finds an antecedent in the laments popular in Tudor ballads and miscellanies. The primary focus of such laments was the predicament of an unchaste woman, usually abandoned, perhaps pregnant; her social predicament is more significant than whether her shame results from seduction or rape. Thomas Howell's (1567–1581) complaint 'To her Lover, that made a conquest of her, and fled, leaving her with child',[1] draws on this lament tradition and, typically, leaves the speaker's volition in the sexual act unclear. Although she describes herself as having been 'by filthy lust beguiled' (l. 54), she laments:

---

1. I have silently modernised the spelling of all quotations from original sources, with the exception of poem titles.

> How could I well deny,
> when needs it must be so:
> Although a shameful I,
> should have a shameless no.
> (1567–1581/1879: ll. 29–32)

Whether defining the sexual act as rape or seduction, the protagonist clearly attributes some blame to the man, exhorting:

> Ponder his filthy deed,
> that left his shame behind.
> (ll. 15–16)

This recalls Mollon's (1996) account of sexual abuse functioning as a projective identification of the shame with the victim, although the 'shame' left behind here is also the child *in utero*.

The difficulty in articulating the difference between rape and seduction, which this poem evidences, reflects contemporary ideas about women's volition. In the late sixteenth century, 'rape' was in transition from being seen as a 'property crime' (the theft of a woman from father or husband) to being seen as sexual violation. The term 'rape' conflated rape, abduction and elopement, with the woman's volition irrelevant. As the concept of female volition developed, however, and the modern definition of rape began to emerge, literary texts increasingly articulated a tension and confusion between these conflicting concepts. The impulse to categorise woman's sexual conduct as either innocent or guilty (based on at least an implicit conception of female volition), thus clashes with an opposing tendency to define all female sexual activity that is not chaste (marital) as illicit. As I have argued elsewhere, the clash between these two impulses gives rise to a common implicit definition of rape in literature of this period as 'forcing a woman to yield' (Catty, 1999: 31).

In an age in which identity and honour for women were always sexual, the development of ideas about rape may be seen as intrinsically related to the developing concept and portrayal of shame. The imperative to women to be chaste was a powerful one. As the definition of rape as a forced violation gradually emerged, rape came to problematise the dichotomy between the chaste and the unchaste. With shame, moreover, being closely bound up with ideas about identity, including sexual identity, the rhetoric of chastity which was powerful at this time may be seen as a rhetoric of shame. The kind of shame represented in the idea of 'shamefastness' (modesty) is represented as a peculiarly feminine virtue in early modern texts. Shame could thus 'refer to the violent loss of chastity, and to the state of mind that would preserve chastity' (Brown, 2004: 6). A woman's shame was supposed to protect her from the shame of unchastity (pre- or extramarital sexual activity) and her husband or father from that of cuckoldry or having a daughter become 'soiled goods'. It thus preserved male property as well as a particular state of mind associated with women.

MIRRORS OF SHAME

The 'female complaint' developed from the earlier lament tradition but was also influenced by the *Mirror for Magistrates* (1559), a collection of tragic complaints uttered by the ghosts of historical figures, which went through multiple editions between 1559 and 1587. The complaint was most popular in the 1590s, but a later example, Barkstead's 'Hiren: or the faire Greek' (1611), attests to the popularity of shame as the focus of the female complaint, when the heroine laments (in a punning allusion to the *Mirror for Magistrates*):

> Too many mirrors have we to behold,
> Of men's inconstancy, and women's shame.
> (1611/1967: 188)

The complaint features a famous mythological or historical female figure, usually returning after her death to lament a downfall which is always in some way sexual. Women raped and committing suicide (Lucrece) and women who kill themselves to avoid rape (Matilda) are featured alongside 'whores' (Helen of Troy, of whom the word 'rape' often means elopement). Mediating these extremes are the complaints of the mistresses of famous men, which present the woman's conduct with varying degrees of ambiguity. These female protagonists may be differentiated by their varying degrees of guilt; but they are united in their shame. The complaint is predicated on the sympathy of the reader for the fallen woman character, a sympathy which seems to be aroused by a fascination with the idea of female sexual shame, distress and dishonour.

Complaints featuring famous mistresses play on an ambivalence about their protagonists' volition, destabilising the distinction between rape and seduction. Even if these women are portrayed as having been raped, their continuing to live on as the men's mistresses undermines the idea of their being victims. In Thomas Churchyard's 'Shores Wife' (1563), Jane Shore uses the language of force to describe her first encounter with Edward IV—'the strong did make the weak to bow' (1563/1991: l. 77)—but undermines this by claiming that she 'agreed the fort he should assault' (l. 84). Samuel Daniel's (1592) 'The Complaint of Rosamond' has the heroine lamenting the political as well as physical power of the king who has shamed her:

> But what? He is my King and may constrain me,
> Whether I yield or not I live defamed:
> The world will think authority did gain me,
> I shall be judged his love, and so be shamed:
> We see the fair condemned, that never gamed.
> And if I yield, tis honourable shame,
> If not, I live disgraced, yet thought the same.
> (1592/1991: ll. 337–43)

The emphasis on the king's power to 'constrain' Rosamond suggests that she fears rape, yet she is depicted as forced into sin both by the 'hand of Lust most undesired' and by her own 'frail flesh'. She laments:

> I saw the shame whereon my flesh was venturing,
> Yet had I not the power for to defend it.
> (ll. 423-4)

Michael Drayton's (1597) version of Rosamond's story displays a similar taste for women as sexual victims and sexually erring. Drawing on the distinction between body and mind that can vindicate raped women, Rosamond says:

> For what my body was enforced to do,
> (Heaven knows) my soul did not consent unto; ...
> Which all the world will to my shame impute
> That I my self did basely prostitute.
> (1597/1991: ll. 33-4, 47-8)

She goes on, however, to lament that Henry has made her 'a monster, both in body and in mind' (l. 174). This notably concrete image unites body and mind in a manner which we may associate with shame.

The complaints dramatise a tension between shame as an affect (the heroine's chief emotion), shamefastness as a feminine ideal and the act of shaming. They also demonstrate an unstable tension between opposed conceptions of chastity as a physical state and as a state of mind, particularly when problematised by rape. The ideological tension surrounding rape has significant implications for the conception of shame, which hinge on a profound ambivalence about whether body and mind reflect one another or are distinct. The relationship between inwardness or interiority and physical display, or between mind and body, was a particularly vexed issue in this period. This has wide-ranging implications for the representation of women's sexual conduct and shame, with female sexuality frequently portrayed as unknowable. While Drayton's Rosamond argues that her soul is not affected by what her body is forced into, she goes on to call herself a monster 'both in body and in mind'. By contrast, Lucrece justifies suicide by arguing that her mind's purity is unaffected by her body's rape; paradoxically, she can only prove this by destroying her body.

This ambiguity about the distinction between mind and body gives rise to two definitions of chastity, both having implications for shame. On the one hand, we find a concrete definition in terms of physical fact: any woman who is neither virgin, faithful wife nor celibate widow is unchaste, regardless of whether the sexual act was consensual or not; she is thus shamed regardless of her volition. On the other hand, we find a more psychological definition, in its emphasis on interiority and the mind: rape is a violation of the body that, because undesired, leaves the woman's mental purity intact. In this psychological context, rape should not produce shame. Yet it is clear that even portrayals of women whose downfall is clearly represented as rape invoke shame as the natural response of the female characters.

I would argue that this is because shame is not only a social emotion, registering social boundaries and mores, and not only an intra-psychic affect, but also a bodily state: not just expressed physiologically but deriving some of its power from the physical. The distinction between mind and body which Rosamond and Lucrece invoke is thus inadequate to liberate them from shame, for the violated body is a shamed body.

THE SPECTACLE OF SHAME

The shamed body is also a viewed body, with display central to the representation of shame. The shamed body becomes a marker for the change of sexual status of its owner: the 'fall' of the woman from virgin or faithful wife to 'whore'. Shamed women in the complaint are held up as spectacle: indeed 'the object[s] as well as the subject[s] of shame' (M Lewis, 1992: 34). Whatever the impulse of the shamed female character to hide her shame (which Shakespeare's Lucrece articulates), the publication of these sexual falls through the poetry is an intrinsic element of the women's shame. Moreover, this shame is often compounded by the theatrical setting of poems in this genre, in which the central female character is usually presented as appearing to the reader/audience to deliver her complaint. The display or disclosure of these female characters may be seen as a voyeuristic act: a public shaming exacerbated when its subject/object is constructed as a woman exhibiting her shame. Exhibitionism and shame, disclosure and secrecy, are thus inscribed in the poems.

Criticism of the gaze has argued that its objectification of women is analogous to rape, and similarly it can surely be seen as a form of shaming. The idea that writing or narrative might be a voyeuristic or shaming act is not anachronistic to the early modern period; on the contrary, prose fiction of the period often exploits the idea. The dangerous exposure effected by narratives about shame is particularly clear in John Trussell's *The First Rape of Faire Hellen* (1595).

Trussell's poem takes a character famous for her adultery or 'rape' (in the sense of abduction/elopement) and has her tell the story of her rape (in the sense of violation) by Theseus when she was a young girl. She first appears in a pose typical of a raped woman, with 'hairs dishevelled, eyes with tears besprent [bespattered]' (Trussell, 1595/1957: l. 21). The poem dramatises a tension between shame as private affect and as public exposure. Hellen's private sense of shame leads her to try to hide after the rape, wishing for darkness and feeling that she cannot 'show my shame' (l. 310): 'shame had sealed my lips with soul's disgrace' (l. 465). But shame is also both a public and a concrete matter, concerning her sexual status. Her nurse comforts her that, because she is too young to conceive, 'thy belly cannot manifest thy wrong' (l. 555) and 'shame hath not charactered upon thy face' (l. 537). She is married off to Menelaus as a cover: 'enfranchised from all fear of shame' (l. 874).

Socially, then, Hellen's rape is concealed and her mental shame is distinguished from the physical and public dimension in this act of covering up. Hellen's urge to 'cover' herself, however, is throughout the poem contrasted with her need to 'complain', both after the rape and after her death, through the poem itself. Even if her rape is 'covered' and kept private, the act of narration publicises and perpetuates her shame. The language of 'disclosure' and 'discovery' permeates the poem. If the root of the word 'shame' means 'to cover oneself', the *act* of shaming is also an uncovering or 'dis-*covery*'. Hellen repeatedly images the shame of public exposure as 'discovery', accusing the sun of shining 'of purpose to discover my disgrace' (l. 214). She laments:

> I cursed the day, the enemy to blame,
> for fear it would my ravishment disclose.
> (ll. 279–80)

The act of narration thus becomes a form of shaming and disclosure. Hellen presents her complaint as uttered under a duress which might come from the poet as much as emotional compulsion:

> That thing did chance which to my endless woe,
> I am *enforced* unto the world to show.
> (ll. 53–4, emphasis added)

At this moment of her rape (enforcement), she calls herself 'the subject of his tyranny' (l. 162): the subject/object of both Theseus's and the poet's acts of literary shaming. That the narrative and the rape may be aligned as shaming acts is also suggested by the poet's use of the language of discovery and disclosure for the rape of Hellen and of her mother, Leda. Theseus rapes Hellen when 'his heart's il-tent [evil intent] he openly discovered'. Leda's rape by Jove in the shape of a swan is effected when he 'discloseth that his feathered plumes; / are God in substance, though a Swan in show' (ll. 625–6). If the female complaint, then, dramatises the shaming of women by presenting women as shaming themselves through the act of complaining, this is a paradox frequently exploited within the poems themselves.

'O UNSEEN SHAME! INVISIBLE DISGRACE!': LUCRECE, SHAME AND SUICIDE

Lucrece's story provides a *locus classicus* not only for the clash between definitions of rape as property crime and as violation, but also for opposed interpretations of shame and guilt. Lucrece, in both Shakespeare's version and his source, William Painter's translation of Livy as *The Palace of Pleasure* (1566), argues that her mind and body are distinct and that she must kill herself to prove that her mind is pure despite her body's pollution by the rape. This has been open to interpretation, however: so much so that Shakespeare's Lucrece refers to it as a 'theme for disputation' (l. 822). St. Augustine (trans. 1610) famously demanded: 'if she be an adulteress, why is she commended? If she be chaste why did she kill her self?' (p. 31). Reading the story in a Christian context in which suicide was sinful, he hypothesised a guilty motive for her suicide: 'she herself gave a lustful consent' (1610: 30).

Augustine's dilemma has been read as manifesting a clash between cultures: Roman culture, in which Lucrece's story originates, has been defined as a 'shame' culture in which a raped woman's shame and loss of reputation were enough to justify her suicide, whereas the emphasis on guilt and conscience in Christian culture led Augustine to infer a guilty motivation (Donaldson, 1982: 21–39). Although this cultural dichotomy is no longer regarded as adequate, it has subsequently been developed to reflect a contrast between cultures which operate by external and internal sanctions, or '(shame-) cultures where morality centres on the self in the world and (guilt-) cultures where morality centres rather on the relationship of the self with others and the law' (Fernie, 2002: 16). Responsibility for the shameful event is irrelevant in classical texts, which evidence little distinction between shame in one's own eyes and shame before the world; in a Christian context, however, shame is an internal matter (ibid: 29). Augustine is attributing to Lucretia an internal sense of shame as having failed in her behaviour by her own standards and God's.

Understanding shame as a global, pervasive sense of pollution or inadequacy goes some way to accounting for suicide as a response to rape. Lucrece's ideological context, however, might equally readily produce interpretations of her suicide as a shameful (escapist) or guilty (reparative) response. As escapist, it might evidence her sense of being globally affected by the violation; indeed, according to the concrete, physical understanding of chastity at the time, the rape made her unchaste whatever her volition. It might equally be read as reparative, however: in this social system, no other way existed for her to right the wrong done to her husband. (By contrast, the rape of virgins was often 'righted' by their marriage to the rapist: a favourite resolution in Jacobean drama (Catty, 1999: 100).) Her story thus bears out the necessity of understanding the cultural context of shame.

Shakespeare's Lucrece finds a context in the diverse catalogue of shamed women of the female complaint genre. *The Rape of Lucrece* (1594) draws on this genre in Lucrece's long lament following the rape, as well as the briefer speech which precedes her suicide. In it, Shakespeare alters his source as far as possible to represent the rape as a forcible violation rather than the 'forcing to yield' presentation found in Painter (Catty, 1999: 66–7) in which the rape is accomplished when 'she vanquished with his terrible and infamous threat. [sic] His fleshly and licentious enterprise, overcame the purity of her chaste heart' (Painter, 1566: f. 5v). The rape in Shakespeare's version is unequivocally violent and personifies shame as the rapist:

> This said, he sets his foot upon the light,
> For light and lust are deadly enemies;
> Shame folded up in blind concealing night,
> When most unseen, then most doth tyrannize.

> The wolf hath seiz'd his prey; the poor lamb cries
> Till with her own white fleece her voice controll'd
> Entombs her outcry in her lips' sweet fold.
> (1594/1960: ll. 673-9)

Shakespeare's poem scrutinises Lucrece's motivation for the suicide that had provoked centuries of clerical 'disputation': motivation that hinges on her expressed shame and guilt. Lucrece's complaint following the rape displays the powerful impulse of the shamed to hide. She feels exposed to the view and censure of 'every eye'; at this point, she seems to have no recourse to the rhetoric that separates mind from body, for she envisages that her eyes will '[en]grave … Upon my cheeks what helpless shame I feel' (ll. 755–6). Thinking of her husband, she cries 'O unseen shame! invisible disgrace!' (l. 827)—the cry encapsulating the paradoxical nature of sexual shame and infamy.

Lucrece's shame is searing; yet she also refers to guilt, blaming herself for entertaining Tarquin as a guest (although 'it had been dishonour to disdain him', l. 844) and implicitly invoking guilt as well as shame in her justification of suicide:

> The remedy indeed to do me good
> Is to let forth this foul, defiled blood.
> Poor hand, why quiver'st thou at this decree?
> Honour thyself to rid me of this shame;
> For if I die my honour lives in thee,
> But if I live thou liv'st in my defame.
> Since thou couldst not defend thy loyal dame,
> And wast afeard to scratch her wicked foe,
> Kill both thyself and her for yielding so.
> (ll. 1028–36)

The image of rape as yielding thus emerges, finally, as Lucrece's own self-accusation. In her dilemma about suicide she calls it 'my poor soul's pollution' (l. 1157), but argues that without it, her soul will 'wither' because of her body's pollution by rape. Her suicide, however, will release her from a shame which here seems emphatically social:

> For in my death I murther shameful scorn,
> My shame is dead, mine honour is new born.
> (ll. 1189–90)

Lucrece's logic is compelling but inconsistent: yet it is precisely its inconsistency which reflects the tension in the conception of shame and rape at this time. The state of being unchaste is always in some sense physical, as images of 'defiled blood' underline. Motivated by both shame and guilt, Lucrece demonstrates through suicide the extent to which shame is still, in 1594, seen as a bodily state.

SHAME AND SHAMING TODAY

In casting our sphere of enquiry back to the poetry of the late sixteenth century, we should not expect to learn any easy lessons about universal psychological truths. Yet while ideas about identity and shame have particular historical and cultural specificity in different periods, the two are clearly associated, with shame being used to work out ideas about selfhood in the early modern period as in the present day. Considering rape, the ultimate act of shaming, challenges our conceptions of shame. (While being raped is widely regarded in Western culture today as 'nothing to be ashamed of', shame is also one of rape's most common psychological corollaries.) Specifically, looking at poems in which rape and other scenarios of sexual shame are narrated exemplifies the extent to which representation and shaming may be intrinsically related.

Representations of women's shame in Elizabethan poetry have clear social and ideological, as well as psychological contexts. As a social emotion as well as a 'self-conscious' one, shame draws on both inner and outer reality. It is appropriate that it is rape—in its uneasy relation to seduction—which is the subject of so many of these poems, for the tensions surrounding representations of rape in its transition from property crime to crime against the person mirror the tensions surrounding shame. Both centre on a clash between a concrete understanding of women's chastity as a physical and social fact and a more symbolic or psychological understanding of chastity as a state of mind.

The complaints link narrative display with shame not just by narrating the shame but also by embodying it in the figure of a female character. This means both that a female body is held up to view and that the portrayal is of a female character shaming *herself*. The degree to which exposure is a key element of shame is thus demonstrated by these female figures, as well as the reliance of culture on visible female bodies. This suggests that there may always be an element of shame or shaming in the display of female bodies. We have seen that identity for women in the early modern period was always sexual and always to a great extent physical. Ideas about shame may be used to work this out because of the dual status of shame as both an emotional and a bodily state: not just in its physiological expression but also in the way in which it is attendant upon certain physical states or experiences. It is perhaps particularly in relation to rape that a more concrete conception of shame comes into play; for the shame attendant upon rape is not wholly containable within an intra-psychic definition of shame. The counterpart to the idea of rape as a form of projective identification of shame (Mollon, 1996: 54) may perhaps be a kind of concrete, bodily experience of shame which is bound up with (sexual) identity and can be seen in heightened form in these texts from an age when chastity was still as much a physical as a mental state.

This begs certain questions. To what extent does the idea of chastity as a physical state endure today? While Western culture no longer invokes it as an ideal, women are still routinely blamed for male sexual behaviour and female bodies are still routinely exhibited as titillation, leaving women in a state of acute awareness of scrutiny and self-scrutiny. Equally, is shame still attendant upon various sexual behaviours, including rape, because of its intrinsic bodily nature, which seems to go beyond merely reflecting shame to being an inherent part of it? The question of the relationship between mind and body also has an enduring valency today, despite no longer being understood in the same terms as in the early modern period. A neuroscientific framework may eventually replace the ideological framework of the sixteenth century in explaining—or at least mapping—this interconnection of the physical and the psychological in states of shame.

Finally, the *act* of shaming is embodied by these poems just as their female characters embody notions of sexual shame. The way in which culture imposes and perpetuates shame is striking. These poems show male poets creating and recreating shamed female characters as a way of embodying ideas about shame, disclosure and publication. Although this had a particular place in late sixteenth-century culture, it also offers an analogy with current literary and popular culture. While there is a familiar lesson here about the reliance of culture on the display of women's bodies, there is also a lesson about what happens to shame when we try to think about or represent it.

It has been suggested that psychotherapy—or specifically the 'therapeutic situation' in which the patient presents him- or herself to the therapist—may be inherently shaming (Mollon, 2002: 133–7). This shaming effect may not simply reside in particular details of setting or stance (such as the therapist's silence, which Mollon cites) or in specific interpretations uttered by the therapist. Given the root of the word shame in the idea of *un*-covering as well as covering—an etymology which reflects a profound interconnection between hiding and exposure or display and concealment which we have seen the female complaint genre exploiting—it may be an inherent meaning of the therapeutic encounter, in which the patient is displayed to a clinician whose role is to uncover or discover their internal world.

Should we also see the complaint poems as attesting to a psychological impulse for confession or lamentation? If so, the gendering of this impulse as female associates it not only with women but also with a specifically sexual shame. The implications of this for the therapeutic situation may apply as much to male as female patients, but the way in which these writers use female characters to embody the interconnections between self-disclosure or lamentation and shame illustrates a profound association between women and shame.

The complaint poets dramatise the inherent shamefulness of the act of complaining. The urge to confess in a therapeutic encounter may itself already contain the patient's own sense of shame. Not only may the therapeutic situation or the clinician's interventions be experienced by the patient as shaming, then, but the act of complaining itself may be experienced as already intrinsically shameful. Given that shame feeds on exposure, this points to a complex interplay between the patient's personal sense of shame in relation to their feelings or history, the sense of shame which may be an inherent part of the confessional impulse, the symbolic shamefulness of the therapeutic situation and the potential for psychological interpretation, as the therapist's act of uncovering, to be an act of shaming. In reflecting our patients to themselves, therapists too may become 'mirrors of shame'.

REFERENCES

Augustine (1610) *Of the Citie of God.* (J Healey, Trans).
Barkstead, W (1967) Hiren: or the faire Greeke. In PW Miller (Ed) *Seven Minor Epics of the English Renaissance.* Gainesville, FL: Scholars' Facsimiles & Reprints. (Original work published 1611)
Bartky, SL (1990) Shame and gender. In SL Bartky *Femininity and Domination: Studies in the phenomenology of oppression* (pp 83–98). New York/London: Routledge.
Brown, G (2004) *Redefining Elizabethan Literature.* Cambridge: Cambridge University Press.
Catty, J (1999) *Writing Rape, Writing Women in Early Modern England: Unbridled speech.* London: Macmillan/New York: St. Martin's Press.
Churchyard, T (1991) Shores wife. In J Kerrigan (Ed) *Motives of Woe: Shakespeare and 'female complaint': A critical anthology* (pp 111–24). Oxford: Clarendon Press. (Original work published 1563)
Daniel, S (1991) The complaint of Rosamond. In J Kerrigan (Ed) *Motives of Woe: Shakespeare and 'female complaint': A critical anthology* (pp 164–90). Oxford: Clarendon Press. (Original work published 1592)
Donaldson, I (1982) *The Rapes of Lucretia: A myth and its transformations.* Oxford: Clarendon Press.
Drayton, M (1991) The epistle of Rosamond to King Henrie the Second. In J Kerrigan (Ed) *Motives of Woe: Shakespeare and 'female complaint': A critical anthology* (pp 192–8). Oxford: Clarendon Press. (Original work published 1597)
Fernie, E (2002) *Shame in Shakespeare.* London/New York: Routledge.
Freud, S (1953) Three essays on sexuality. In J Strachey (Ed) *Standard Edition of the Complete Works of Freud, Vol 7.* London: Hogarth Press. (Original work published 1905)
Freud, S (1964) New introductory lectures on psycho-analysis. In J Strachey (Ed) *Standard Edition of Complete Works of Freud, Vol 22* (pp 3–182). London: Hogarth Press. (Original work published 1933.)
Gilbert, P (2002) Body shame: A biopsychosocial conceptualisation and overview, with treatment implications. In P Gilbert & J Miles (Eds) *Body Shame: Conceptualisation, Research and Treatment* (pp 3–54). Hove/New York: Brunner-Routledge.
Howell, T (1879) To her Louer, that made a conquest of her, and fled, leauing her with childe. In AB Grosart (Ed) *Thomas Howell's Poems (1567–81).* Manchester: Occasional Issues of Unique or Very Rare Books. (Original Work published 1567–1581)
Levy, R & Rosaldo, MS (Eds) (1983) Special Issue Devoted to Self and Emotion. *Ethos 11*(3).
Lewis, HB (1971) *Shame and guilt in neurosis.* New York: International Universities Press.
Lewis, M (1992) *Shame: The exposed self.* New York/Oxford: Macmillan, Free Press.
Mirror for Magistrates (1559).
Mollon, P (1996) *Multiple Selves, Multiple Voices: Working with trauma, violation and dissociation.* New York/Chichester: Wiley.
Mollon, P (2002) *Shame and Jealousy: The hidden turmoils.* London/New York: Karnac.
Oxford English Dictionary (1989) (2nd edn). Oxford: Oxford University Press.
Painter, W (1566) *The Palace of Pleasure.*
Parker, R (2003) Body hatred. *British Journal of Psychotherapy, 19* (4), 447–64.
Pines, M (1995) The universality of shame: A psychoanalytic approach. *British Journal of Psychotherapy, 11* (3), 346–57.

Shakespeare, W (1960/1985) The rape of Lucrece. In FT Prince (Ed) *The Poems*. London/New York: Methuen. (Original work published 1594)

Tangney, JP (1995) Shame and guilt in interpersonal relationships. In JP Tangney & KW Fischer (Eds) *Self-Conscious Emotions: The psychology of shame, guilt, embarrassment, and pride* (pp 114–39). New York/London: Guilford Press.

Trussell, J (1957) The first rape of faire Hellen. MA Shaaber (Ed) as The first rape of faire Hellen by John Trussell, *Shakespeare Quarterly* (1957), *viii*, 407–48. (Original work published 1595)

Wall, W (1993) *The Imprint of Gender: Authorship and publication in the English Renaissance*. Ithaca, NY/London: Cornell University Press.

Wurmser, L (1981) *The Mask of Shame*. Northvale, NJ/London: Jason Aronson (reprinted 1994).

Acknowledgements

Thanks are due to Connie Geyer and Rosie Parker for their insightful comments on this paper; and to the organisers and audience of the Association for Medical Humanities annual conference, King's College, London, at which this paper was presented in September 2006.

CHAPTER 9

SYMPTOMS IN SOCIETY
THE CULTURAL SIGNIFICANCE OF FATIGUE IN VICTORIAN BRITAIN

Christopher D. Ward

INTRODUCTION

The medical model of illness encourages us to think of symptoms as products of disease, but symptoms also have interpersonal meaning: complaining of pain or itching or deafness or shortness of breath confers social significance on behaviours such as wincing, or scratching, or social withdrawal. Conversely, illness behaviour may be constitutive of symptoms; thus, we are reluctant to give credence to a description of pain unless we observe pain behaviour. Viewing symptoms as interpersonal phenomena shifts the focus towards their social context. In the case of depression, an interpersonal or systemic approach has been shown to be therapeutically useful at the level of immediate relationships (Jones & Asen, 2000). A still broader view of depression takes account of factors such as gender, power, economics and so on. Could the same be said of a physical symptom? My purpose here is to show how cultural influences might have influenced the expression of fatigue as a symptom in the nineteenth century. I will end by considering what parallels might be drawn between neurasthenia, a late nineteenth-century diagnosis, and its modern equivalent, the chronic fatigue syndrome (CFS).

In late Victorian medicine, neurasthenia was described as a disease entity characterised by fatigue ('asthenia', lack of energy) together with 'disturbed sleep ... vague pains ... and various phenomena referable to the vaso-motor and sympathetic systems' (Savill, 1906). There was 'a peculiar mental state, and ... dyspepsia' (Ballet, 1911). Many of these features, together with intolerance of lights and sounds, were summed up as 'irritable weakness' (Savill, 1906; Ballet, 1911). The term 'neurasthenia' was introduced in the 1870s in both America and Britain. Prior to then, similar symptoms had not been differentiated from hysteria; neurasthenia was considered to be primarily a disease of men, whereas the reverse was true of hysteria.

In what follows I will consider two intersecting cultural strands which are related to the emergence of neurasthenia as a disease concept: first, contemporaneous scientific concepts of energy and fatigue, and second, the themes of weariness, rest and oblivion in literature and religion. The intention is not to 'explain away' neurasthenia. Instead, I wish to build a picture of a Victorian patient whose cultural milieu has the effect of contributing to his distress as well as constraining the means of expression available to him and to his doctor. Conceivably, the patient with CFS is in a similar predicament in our own time.

BIOLOGICAL FATIGUE

Neurobiological theorising—much of it purely speculative—directly or indirectly supplied clinicians and patients with explanatory stories around which fatigue could come to be seen as a medical illness. Two principal sources were Alexander Bain and Herbert Spencer: Bain was the most influential writer on the science of brain and mind prior to Spencer, whose views became the post-Darwinian orthodoxy. One of their major projects was to describe the energetics of bodies and brains in physical terms. This paved the way for physicians to claim that neurasthenia was a neurologically determined lack of energy.

In the period leading up to the advent of neurasthenia, biological thinking concerned itself with six relevant concepts: (1) energy as a property of tissues and organs; (2) nerve force, recalling Newtonian mechanics; (3) electrical batteries and currents as sources of nervous energy; (4) chemistry as a model both for the blood-born supply of energy and for the deleterious effects of waste products; (5) the economic model of energy management; and (6) the equation of mind with brain, so that psychology was represented as 'mental physiology'.

1. FATIGUE IN TISSUES AND ORGANS

As a legacy of pre-modern vitalism, body tissues were often considered to have intrinsic energies. 'Tone' was represented as a general property of living tissues and throughout the nineteenth century 'tonics' continued to be provided as means of restoring tone not only to the muscles but also to the nerves. Irritability, advocated by John Brown in the previous century, was a positive attribute of tissues. According to Sinclair (1818), exhaustion was due to a loss of natural irritability and called for absolute rest, 'until the irritable principle is again accumulated, and nature restores by sleep, that vital energy which the body had lost by its former exertions' (p. 305).

In mid-century, fatigue was still considered to affect organs and tissues as well as the organism as a whole. Nervous exhaustion was a tissue disorder, according to Bain, and the benefits of rest and stimulants were due to 'a change wrought on the substance of the nerve tissue'. In a clinical context, general prostration could be described as 'the state of asthenia, or depressed nerve-power' (Hovell, 1867: 13). It was but a small step from this statement of 1867 to the crystallisation in the 1870s of the concept of 'neurasthenia' as a *neurological* disorder. In our own times, the medical formulation of CFS ('myalgic encephalomyelitis' or 'encephalopathy') implies disease of central nervous tissues—including, but not exclusively the brain.

Another ill-defined network of ideas concerned the notion of semen as a source of life force. Spermatorrhoea was an entity advocated mainly but not exclusively by quacks. Loss of sperm through masturbation or nocturnal emissions was the putative cause of many ills, including impotence (Mason, 1994). General debility of the organism was often held to be the result of sexual excess and by the end of the century many orthodox medical authorities recognised the category of sexual neurasthenia. Freud, in 1896, pronounced that:

Pure neurasthenia, which after it has been differentiated from anxiety neurosis presents a monotonous clinical picture (exhaustion, sense of pressure on the head, flatulent dyspepsia, constipation, spinal paraesthesias, sexual weakness, etc), admits of only two specific aetiological factors, excessive onanism and spontaneous emissions. (Freud, 1924: 146)

2. NEUROMECHANICS

In an age of mechanization, the nervous system was viewed less as an information processor than as a source and regulator of energy. Bain considered that 'when the brain is in action, there is some transmission of nerve power' (Bain, 1855: 61); '[a] system of intercommunication and transmission of power is … an essential part of the bodily and mental structure' (ibid: 58). Herbert Spencer, a Derby railway engineer before he became the unchallenged doyen of social scientists and psychologists, wrote about nervous pressure and compared cerebral action to a steam engine, with 'the arrival of the piston at a certain point … necessarily accompanied by the opening of a valve serving to admit the steam which will drive the piston in the reverse direction' (Spencer, 1899: 430). Clinicians translated these ideas directly into interpretations of neurasthenia:

[T]his sensation of fatigue, this feeling of heaviness in the body, this need of making efforts in order to walk, to go upstairs, or to stand up, this emptiness in the head, which gives the impression that one is about to faint, but which never goes so far, this distressing need of recruiting one's strength, this whole group of symptoms that characterises nervous exhaustion, all these are based on fixed laws which are laws of mechanics. (Ballet, 1911: 139)

3. BIO-ELECTRICITY

Today, the discharge and recharging of batteries is a familiar image for fatigue and recuperation. Applying the same image to neurasthenia a hundred years ago, Savill wrote: 'Just as a faradic battery, after continuous use, gradually becomes weaker … and then after a rest becomes restored again, so does nervous force require periods of intermission for recuperation' (Savill, 1906: 68). Here, electricity is not so much an analogy as a possible model for the still obscure nature of 'nervous force'; similar ambivalence can be traced to Spencer, writing that 'we must regard the entire nervous system as at all times discharging itself'. Disturbing any part of the nervous system produced 'conspicuous emissions of force' (Spencer, 1899: 93).

4. BIOCHEMISTRY

For Spencer, chemistry was a possible key to the mystery of nerve force, which he pictured as 'waves of molecular change, that chase one another rapidly through nerve … fibres' (Spencer, 1899: 95). 'The quantity of molecular motion locked up in a nerve-centre, is measured by the contained quantity of unstable nerve-matter' (Spencer, 1899: 86). There was an intimate relationship between production of nerve force and blood supply: 'blood rich in the constituents of nerve substance, renders possible a great evolution nerve-force' (Spencer, 1899: 74). A feeble heart would produce diminished 'nervous power'; conversely '[when] a nerve-centre is highly charged with arterial blood ... [it] evolves more than ordinary amounts of force' (Spencer, 1899: 73).

Ballet demonstrated the use of these ideas to depict neurasthenia as 'an intimate derangement of the nutrition of the nerve elements; these nerve elements, it is thought, have increased difficulty in recruiting their exhausted energy, and no longer accumulate to the same degree as in health the force that they discharge' (Ballet, 1911: 2).

5. THE BODILY ECONOMY

The Newtonian concept of conservation of energy was a basis for integrating mechanical, electrical and chemical concepts in an economic model of organic function, where the production and consumption of nervous force was balanced. Thus, according to Bain, 'the conducting power of a nerve fibre is a wasting operation, one that draws upon the vitality of the fibre, and causes the necessity for times of rest and a copious supply of nourishment' (Bain, 1855: 121). Today, therapeutic concepts of 'pacing' encourage CFS patients to conceive of energy as a finite store which must be carefully husbanded. In a similar way, neurasthenia was seen as a breakdown in the body's energy economy: 'Many neurasthenics have the ability to spend in a very short time all the reserve energy of their CNS and an instant later they become powerless' (Lagrange, cited in Creuzet, 1917). Bain provided an antecedent for this idea: 'The ordinary and enduring currents of activity can be converted into an extraordinary discharge of short duration at the expense of the future' (Bain, 1859: 34).

6. THE MENTAL PHYSIOLOGY OF FATIGUE

In neurasthenia, mental manifestations were no less prominent than physical symptoms, and a crucial step in the development of a scientific rationale for neurasthenia was the extension of energy ideas to psychological processes. In the first place, each of the conceptual frameworks considered above had a psychological dimension. Thus, Bain connected the mechanical actions of muscles to psychic equivalents: 'A movement, whether real or ideal, is mentally known as a definite expenditure of energy in some special muscle or muscles' (Bain, 1875: 148). Electrical concepts suggested the idea of currents and these were fundamental to mental function ('no currents, no mind', Bain, 1855: 62); for Bain, currents conveyed force, not information. Bain presumed 'that feelings of exhilaration and of depression are connected with the circulation of the blood and the nourishment of the tissues' (Bain, 1875: 32). Similarly, Spencer pronounced that 'general abundance of blood is a cause of emotional exaltation' and that 'depletion is a cause of apathy'. The intensity of emotion increased with increasing blood supply, 'notwithstanding the waste that has taken place'; however, 'a diminished capacity for emotion inevitably follows each gush of emotion' (Spencer, 1899: Vol 1, 121–2). The concept was of a 'quantifiable economy of feeling energies' and cognitive capacity was similarly constrained by competing demands of the energy economy:

> When muscular effort is suddenly pushed to excess, say by running a long way at full speed or by climbing a mountain till forced to desist by want of breath, the power of thinking is appreciably diminished. A very strong emotion makes such a draught on the supply of nervous fluid as to incapacitate the intellect throughout. (Spencer, 1899: 595–6)

At the turn of the century, in the heyday of neurasthenia, the standard physiological account of fatigue in Britain was a translation of Mosso's monograph (1904), which presented a similar range of models. Principles of energy conservation remained central. The key regulator of both muscular and cerebral energy was blood supply, which conveyed nutrients, removed waste products and thereby constrained the energy economy; this was the link that connected mental to physical fatigue.

Much of the writing about the dependence of mental and muscular energy on blood supply could be read in modern terms as an account of how the brain and the body were supplied with fuel; in the twentieth-first century energy is often a synonym for fuel and fatigue can be conceptualised as fuel depletion. There is then an implicit body–mind dualism which leaves a question unanswered: if the brain and the muscles are the engines of action, what drives the engine, what kind of energy does the driver require, and how could mental fatigue be a coherent concept? The roots of this dualism are implied in Mosso, who had a modern view of nerves as communication media like telegraph wires; the locus for fatigue was not the wires themselves, but the brain and the muscles conceived as 'two telegraph offices' (Mosso, 1904: 281). Brain fatigue must be exhaustion of the ability to process information rather than the failure of motivational force. Similarly, Deschamps was at pains to distinguish disorders of 'distribution' from disorders of 'production' of energy (Deschamps, 1909: 47).

These ideas marked a new phase in neuroscience; fifty years earlier, Bain's model had been less dualistic. His 'currents' were currents of activity not information (see above). His model of nervous force was, at root, a model of voluntary action. 'After every night's repose, and after the nourishment of a meal, the active organs are charged with power ready to explode in any direction' (Bain, 1859: 112). Selecting a course of action was a question of managing the energy economy: 'wherever two present sensations [take] opposite courses, there is an experiment upon the relative strength of the two' (Bain, 1859: 134). The sensation of effort arose from 'muscular pain joined to the pain of the conflict of motives' (Bain, 1875: 362). Energy for action entailed overcoming 'languor' but energies were liable to 'collapse' before a task was accomplished (Bain, 1859: 77). 'A jaded horse needs more spurring' (Bain, 1875: 348) but:

> The time comes when no amount of pain will procure a single muscular contraction. The inability is now physical and not moral. That condition of spontaneous overflow indispensable as a preliminary in the formation of the innumerable links of voluntary control ... according as the nervous batteries grow feeble, the prompting calls have to be increased, until at a certain pitch of depletion there is a total incapacity of evolving any further quota of power. (Bain, 1859: 125)

These ideas could readily be translated into a psychophysical account of neurasthenia as a collapse of the nervous system in response to excessive external pressure. Victorian life was inconvenient, cold and disease-prone and people worked hard. The stress of modern life—'over pressure', or in the French literature 'surmenage'—was commonly invoked as the primary cause of neurasthenia:

> Perhaps the chief cause of the increase in the disease among the upper and great middle classes ... [is] the greater pace at which we live. The introduction of railways and other improved means of communication, the large proportional increase in the town dwellers, as compared with the rural folk, all tend largely to increase the rate at which life is carried on. This is especially so in the metropolis, where nearly every other person you meet seems to be trying to get two days' work into one. The insufficient air and light and the forms of our great cities are also, without doubt, potent factors in the increase of neurasthenia. (Savill, 1906: 111)

Like Bain's jaded horse, the victim of 'over pressure' progressed '[from] simple fatigue to exhaustion, from exhaustion to collapse, from collapse to death' (Richardson, 1879: 120).

MORAL FATIGUE

Writers such as Bain, Spencer and Savill sought physiological accounts for the effects of modern life, but late Victorian poetry and religious thinking were also concerned with the themes of fatigue and weariness. The concept of energy resonated with key Victorian values such as manliness, courage and entrepreneurial spirit. Spencer, for one, was personally implicated in this. His theoretical accounts of energy and fatigue connected on the one hand with his own extraordinary productivity and on the other hand with the listless, neurasthenic state described by his biographers and in his autobiography (Spencer, 1904; Thomson, 1906). Bain had a personal connection with fatigue through his friend John Stuart Mill, who was troubled by episodes of malaise (Bain, 1882).

POETIC AND RELIGIOUS VISIONS OF WEARINESS AND OBLIVION

In the latter half of the nineteenth century there was a flowering (if that is the word) of references to weariness in poems and hymns. There was inner weariness, typified by Matthew Arnold: 'Weary of myself, and sick of asking | What I am, and what I ought to be';[1] and by Christina Rossetti: 'God strengthen me to bear myself; | That heaviest weight of all to bear, | Inalienable weight of care'.[2] Then there was the weariness of doubt, grief and remorse, often to be found in Swinburne: 'Grieve thee? art thou soul-sick till day be done, | and weary till day rises? Is thine heart | full of dead things as mine is?';[3] 'With weary days thou

---
1. 'Self-Dependence' (Matthew Arnold, 1896: 255).
2. 'Who Shall Deliver Me?' (Christina Rossetti, 1904: 238).
3. 'Tristram of Lyonesse: Iseult at Tinagel' (Swinburne, 1904: 79).

shalt be clothed and fed, | And wear remorse of heart for thine attire'.[4] Weariness resulted from the ceaseless struggle of life itself, prompting Matthew Arnold's lament: 'With aching hands and bleeding feet | We dig and heap, lay stone on stone; | We bear the burden and the heat | Of the long day, and wish 'twere done'.[5]

For a Christian such as Christina Rossetti, life's moral struggle made one 'weary in well-doing'. 'Day after day I plod and moil: | But, Christ my God, when will it be | That I may let alone my toil | And rest with Thee?'.[6] The image of moral fatigue was absorbed into the very heart of Victorian Christianity. A key text was Matthew 11.28 for which the *Good News Bible* (1974) gives a typical modern translation: 'Come to me, all you who are tired from carrying heavy loads, and I will give you rest'. Neither tiredness nor rest are central to the pre-Victorian (seventeenth-century) translations of the biblical verse, which had been rendered in the Book of Common Prayer as: 'Come unto me all that travail and are heavy laden, and I will refresh you'; the King James version was: 'Come unto me, all ye that labour and are heavy laden and I will give you rest', where rest is a reward for a good day's work rather than an antidote to fatigue. In contrast, many Victorian hymns substituted 'weary' for hard work, and 'rest' for 'refresh'.[7] J.M. Neale's hymn is typical: 'Art thou weary, art thou languid, Art thou sore distrest? "Come to me" saith One, "and coming Be at rest!"'.[8] Here, not only is the moral tone Victorian but so also are the aesthetics of languor and weariness, as though Christ's mission on earth was to combat ennui.

The pattern of life for late Victorian Christianity is presented in Edmeston's hymn depicting Jesus' temptation in the wilderness: 'Lone and dreary, faint and weary, Through the desert thou didst go'.[9] Rest was elevated to the highest value: 'Day after day I plod and moil: But, Christ my God when will it be That I may let alone my toil And rest with thee?';[10] 'In the weary hours of sickness, In the times of grief and pain, When we feel our mortal weakness, When all human help is vain: By thy mercy Oh deliver us good Lord'.[11] Victorians appeared to be looking heavenward for rest but many perceived the 'struggling, task'd morality' of Christianity as part of life's 'over pressure'. Nature, not God, speaks for peace in Matthew Arnold's 'Morality': 'There is no effort on my brow [says Nature] – | I do not strive, I do not weep; | I rush with the swift spheres and glow | In joy, and when I will, I sleep'.[12]

---

4. 'A Ballad of Burdens' (Swinburne, 1884: 142).
5. 'Morality' (Arnold, 1896: 256).
6. 'Weary in Well-doing' (Rossetti, 1904: 242).
7. All references are to *Hymns Ancient & Modern Revised* (1950). For example: 'O love that wilt not let me go, I rest my weary soul in thee' (A&MR, 359; G Matheson); 'I heard the voice of Jesus say, "Come unto me and rest; Lay down, thou weary one, lay down Thy head upon my breast." I came to Jesus as I was, Weary and worn and sad; I found in him a resting place, And he has made me glad' (A&MR, 351; H Bonar); 'Come unto me, ye weary, And I will give you rest' (A&MR, 350; W Chatterton Dix); 'Come, weary souls, for Jesus bids you come … And laden souls, by thousands meekly stealing, Kind Shepherd, turn their weary steps to thee … Rest comes at length: though life be long and dreary' (A&MR, 354; FW Faber).
8. JM Neale: 'Art Thou Weary' (A&MR, 348).
9. J Edmeston: 'Lead Me Heavenly Father Lead Me' (A&MR, 311).
10. JJ Cummins: 'Jesus Lord of Life and Glory' (A&MR, 321).
11. 'Morality' (Arnold, 1896: 256).
12. Ibid: 256.

The corollary of the Victorians' fatigue-saturated sensibility was a longing for oblivion. This had been a relatively innocent fancy in Keats' ode to the nightingale[13] but as weariness bore down later in the century, so the death wish became darker: 'Ah yet would God that stems and roots were bred | Out of my weary body and my head, | That sleep were sealed upon me with a seal, | And I were as the least of all his dead';[14] '.... her heart was tired, tired, | And now they let her be';[15] 'Sleep, let me sleep, for my pain wearies me'.[16] No clearer demonstration could be found of the pervasiveness of this theme than its appearance in Bain's neurologically orientated treatise *Emotions and the Will*, where he writes of 'the total loss of freshness and tone through the entire substance of the nervous system, the final triumph of ennui: "I am aweary, aweary, | O God that I were dead"' (Bain, 1859: 270).[17]

THE MORAL DIMENSION OF MEDICAL FATIGUE

Bain's physiological account of brain fatigue shaded imperceptibly into a description of personal or moral collapse: when one's nervous batteries were sapped of willpower one became irresolute and ineffectual. Writing prior to the popularity of neurasthenia, Richardson observed such effects in those who chose a life of pleasure at the expense of the brain's need for sleep. They developed 'a mental feebleness and imbecility which end in complete failure of mental power. Doubt and hesitation are succeeded by distrust, distrust by fear, which sound sleep so beneficently ministers' (Richardson, 1879: 437). These were the selfsame psychic factors which Allbutt enshrined in his textbook account of neurasthenia: 'lost interest in life, self-centred ... inattentive, from sheer lack of power of application, of mental attack and endurance ... loss of volition, of self-control, and of initiative ... loss of control' (Allbutt, 1899: 139). Descriptions such as these seem to provide a neurological basis for moral or sociological disengagement. Allbutt's patients, one might say, manifested anomie in declining their responsibilities and acting on groundless, impulsive decisions. This was the wanton attitude which Bain had described: 'painful exhaustion' produced 'collapsed features, restlessness, fretting, and melancholy' and in response to these '[t]he action suggested is usually something quite extravagant and misplaced' (Bain, 1859: 270).

In the passage just quoted, Bain's psychophysiological account of 'ennui' was couched in terms familiar at the time, and prefigured neurasthenia. According to Creuzet, the neurasthenic's ennui was based on his 'notion of moral and physical inferiority' but its origin was 'slowing of the vital movement'; ennui thus had a cerebral origin (Creuzet, 1917: 63). In the opposite causal direction, Ballet wrote that 'depressing emotions in

---

13. '[F]or many a time | I have been half in love with easeful Death ... Now more than ever seems it rich to die, | To cease upon the midnight with no pain, | While thou art pouring forth thy soul abroad | In such an ecstasy!'. Ode to a Nightingale. *The Complete Poetical Works of John Keats*. Edited with an introduction and textual notes by H Buxton Forman. (Keats, 1907: 230 stanza VI).
14. 'Laus Veneris' (Swinburne, 1884: 15).
15. 'Requiescat' (Arnold, 1896: 21).
16. 'Looking Forward' (Rossetti, 1904: 293).
17. Bain quotes from Alfred Lord Tennyson: 'Mariana' (Tennyson, 1878).

reality constitute a source of fatigue, a cause of wear and tear to the nervous centres, far more powerful than brain-work' (Ballet, 1911: 19). In the present context the question of the relationship between neurasthenia and depression is of secondary interest and it is sufficient to note that we arrive here at an intersection between scientific models of fatigue and constructions of weariness and ennui which permeated Victorian culture during the same period.

SOCIAL FATIGUE

There are hazards in viewing illnesses as metaphor, as Susan Sontag (1983) recognised, but in the case of neurasthenia there is a persuasive case for linking symptoms and cultural meanings. Several related factors could have contributed to the metaphorical significance of fatigue in the nineteenth century. Weariness, ennui and the desire for oblivion became increasingly important themes towards the end of the century and one can see how the symptom of fatigue might have resonated with its cultural context. In the first place there were the physical manifestations and social upheavals associated with industrialisation. Much poetic weariness could be read as a romantic reaction to industrial capitalism and its attendant stresses, and Rabinbach suggested that neurasthenia 'reflected an anxiety about body and self in the face of modernity's demands' (cited in Killen, 2006: 11).

The soul as well as the body was under threat during this period. Modernity was posing new problems for Christianity even before the cataclysm of evolutionary theory, and this might have been one reason why the Christian life was more and more frequently represented as a wearisome business. The presentation of fatigue as a symptom might have been a substitute for more direct expression of moral or spiritual confusions. As in hysteria, the medicalisation of fatigue could have had the effect of neutralising potentially subversive positions.

Gender was a touchstone for many of the tensions latent in Victorian society. Hysteria has been seen as a form of coded communication used by women to articulate their powerlessness (Showalter, 1987, 1997) and one might speculate that the neurasthenic state could have represented the predicaments of men. Oppenheim (1991) described a transformation of masculinity across the century. Emotional expressiveness and aestheticism were more acceptable early in the century than later, when there was greater emphasis on action and achievement. According to Killen there were fears that the fatiguing effects of 'over-civilization' would lead to 'un-manning'.

NEURASTHENIA AND CHRONIC FATIGUE SYNDROME

Given the cultural resonances of fatigue in the nineteenth century it would be tempting to conclude that neurasthenia was a product of its time, bearing no relationship to a biological process. However, the symptoms of neurasthenia were not uniquely linked to their specific social context. As Wessely (1991) suggested, the core aspects of neurasthenia are reproduced in the modern chronic fatigue syndrome (CFS). In CFS, as in neurasthenia, fatigue is associated with sleep disturbance, memory impairment, sore throat, non-specific pains, intolerance of lights and sounds, and abdominal symptoms (Reeves et al, 2003; Wessely, Hotopf & Sharpe, 1998; Shepherd, 1999). Similarities between neurasthenia and CFS seem to legitimise neurasthenia as a clinical diagnosis. Further support for a biological rather than a sociological explanation comes from epidemiological evidence showing that the symptoms of CFS can be demonstrated in a wide variety of communities across the world (Reeves, 2005).

Might not both neurasthenia and CFS be easier to explain in biological than in cultural terms, given the many contrasts between nineteenth-century and twenty-first-century social conditions?

THE REALITY OF NEURASTHENIA AND CFS

The reality of neurasthenia seems to have been continuously questioned (Oppenheim, 1991; Shorter, 1992). According to a prevalent view (which Sir Clifford Allbutt was vigorously contesting), neurasthenia was 'in part a sham and in part a figment of complacent physicians'; '[a] mere hotchpot—[a] limbo into which the odds and ends of unconsidered neurotic trifles are to be thrust' (Allbutt, 1899: 137). Patients with CFS are in a similar situation. Their concern is to establish CFS as an authentic, physically based illness. In the nineteenth and early twentieth centuries no specific physical markers of neurasthenia were found although the search was intensive. Modern diagnostic technologies have been no more successful in the case of CFS, leaving open the question of whether either condition could represent a valid disease category. The 'reality' of CFS is currently an emotive issue on the one hand for affected individuals and patient-led organisations, and on the other hand for sceptics. As I write, the Prime Minister is being presented with a petition proclaiming that 'ME is real'.[18]

Both sides of the debate about CFS use the same physical frame of reference as was used in connection with neurasthenia. For the Victorian physicians, 'real' diseases had a biological basis and symptoms could only derive meaning from the patient's body, never from his personal or social world: 'Medical men deal not with words but with things' (Riadore, 1843: 41). One source of anxiety for patients, and a reason for their preference for the diagnosis of neurasthenia, was the shame attached to psychiatric diagnoses: '[t]he word neurasthenia has been a great comfort to doctors and to the friends of patients. Not unnaturally these friends dread the term insanity, and rejoice to hear that the patient is only suffering from neurasthenia' (Savage, 1911, cited in Shorter, 1992: 223). The only remaining possibility was to be consigned to the limbo of 'neurotic trifles', with the implication that the symptoms were trivial and essentially self-produced. No wonder patients with neurasthenia sought a medical explanation for their symptoms: things seemed safer than words.

In discussing the 'realness' of CFS the defining criteria are again things, not words;

---

18. We the undersigned petition the Prime Minister to get the Health Service and medical profession to accept the WHO classification of ME/CFS as an organic neurological disorder and not as a psychosocial syndrome <http://petitions.pm.gov.uk/ME-is-real/> (verified 29 November 2007).

the polar concepts are biological processes such as viral infection, intoxications, nutritional deficiencies and so on, and CFS is real if these are real, but not otherwise (see Shepherd, 1999). If a physical abnormality such as thyroid deficiency is found, a blood result has replaced a symptom as the defining feature and 'realness' is assured. If not, then CFS may be suggested as a 'diagnosis of exclusion'—exclusion, the patient assumes, from the realm of the real.

Writing as a clinician, it is clear to me that CFS produces real distress and disability, whatever the mechanism might be. It seems likely that this was equally true of neurasthenia. Sir Clifford Allbutt was therefore right to insist that neurasthenia should not have been dismissed as a 'trifle'. The contentious issue for neurasthenia, as for CFS, was its status within medicine. As Berrios' work demonstrates (Berrios, 1996), the history of symptoms is an aspect of the history of ideas as well as of the history of diseases. Neurasthenia occupied a sort of Gaza Strip, an unstable border zone between medicine and psychiatry. In the pre-Freudian era there was no third space within which a person weighed down with functional symptoms could legitimately seek professional help. Efforts made today to secure the authenticity of CFS extend across the same territory, still untainted by psychotherapeutic concepts, as though Freud had never existed. Psychological distress is admitted as a secondary phenomenon but not as a legitimate reason for feeling ill.

THE MEANINGS OF SYMPTOMS

The crucial question for people with CFS, as for neurasthenia, is the validity and credibility of symptoms. A symptom is made of words, not things: it is a speech act with discursive significance. We can distinguish not only between fatigue as a bodily process and fatigue as a subjective feeling (Berrios, 1990), but also between fatigue as an inner experience and fatigue as a social signifier. The interpersonal meaning of a symptom derives from understandings established between an individual and an audience: not just between a patient and a physician but also, say, between a child and a mother. Prevailing ideas (discourses) always constrain the types of subjective experiences or dispositions which are available for individuals to communicate to one another. I have tried to show something of the rich pattern of meanings associated with words for fatigue in the nineteenth century.

To achieve a biopsychosocial synthesis, and to register the cultural context of a symptom such as fatigue, we need to show how symptoms can be both biologically based *and* meaningful. Perhaps Freud's most important innovation was to take the content of symptoms seriously, leading not only to psychoanalysis but also to other forms of psychotherapy in functional disorders (see for example Dubois, 1909 and André-Thomas, 1912). Such approaches were (and still are) focused on individuals. A cultural perspective might prompt us to extend our attention beyond the intrapersonal sphere to the interpersonal or systemic aspect of symptoms, opening up radically different therapeutic avenues. Applying what Mills (1959) called a 'sociological imagination' to fatigue in its modern forms would enable us to be aware not only of 'personal troubles of milieu' but also of 'public issues of social structure'. When considering neurasthenia from a historical perspective, 'issues of social structure' are in the foreground while 'personal troubles' are obscured from view. In our clinical encounters with functional disorders such as CFS, the reverse is true.

REFERENCES

Allbutt TA (1899) Neurasthenia. In TA Allbutt (Ed) *A System of Medicine, Vol 8* (pp 134–63). London: Macmillan.
André-Thomas (1912) *Psychothérapie*. Paris: Librairie J-B Baillière.
Arnold, M (1896) *Poetical Works of Matthew Arnold*. London: Macmillan.
Bain, A (1855) *The Senses and the Intellect*. London: John W Parker.
Bain, A (1859) *The Emotions and the Will*. London: John W Parker & Son.
Bain, A (1875) *Mental and Moral Science: Part First: Psychology and history of philosophy*. London: Longman's Green.
Bain, A (1882) *John Stuart Mill: A criticism, with personal recollections*. London: Longman's & Co.
Ballet, G (1911) *Neurasthenia*. London: Henry Kimpton.
Berrios, G (1990) Feelings of fatigue and psychopathology: A conceptual history. *Comprehensive Psychiatry, 31*, 140–51.
Berrios, G (1996) *The History of Mental Symptoms*. Cambridge: Cambridge University Press.
Creuzet, P (1917) *Les Misères des Neurasthéniques*. Paris: Vigot Frères.
Deschamps, A (1909) *Les Maladies de l'Energie. Les asthénies générales, epuisements, insuffisances, inhibitions. Clinique – Thérapeutique*. Paris : Felix Alcan.
Dubois, P (1909) *Pathogeny of the Neurasthenic States* (EG Richards, Trans). Edinburgh: William Green.
Freud, S (1924) Heredity and the aetiology of the neuroses. In S Freud *Collected Papers, Vol 1* (J Riviere, Trans) (pp 138–54). New York: International Psychoanalytical Press. (Originally published in Revue Neurologique, 1896.)
Good News Bible (1976) London: Collins.
Hovell, D de Berdt (1867) *On Pain and Other Symptoms Connected with Hysteria*. London: J Churchill.
Hymns Ancient & Modern Revised (1950). London: Clowes.
Jones, E & Asen E (2000) *Systemic Couple Therapy and Depression*. London/New York: Karnak.
Keats, J (1907) *The Complete Poetical Works of John Keats*, H Buxton Forman (Ed). London: Henry Frowde, Oxford University Press.
Killen, A (2006) *Berlin Electropolis: Shock, nerves, and German modernity*. Berkeley, CA: University of California Press.
Mason, M (1994) *The Making of Victorian Sexuality*. Oxford: Oxford University Press.
Mills, C Wright (1959) *The Sociological Imagination*. Oxford/New York: Oxford University Press.
Mosso, A (1904) *Fatigue*. (M Drummond & WR Drummond, Trans). London: Swan Sonnenschein.
Oppenheim, J (1991) *Shattered Nerves*. New York/Oxford: Oxford University Press.
Reeves, WC (2005) Epidemiology of chronic fatigue syndrome. National Conference of CFS/ME Investment Programme, London.
Reeves, WC, Lloyd, A, Vernon, SD et al (2003) Identification of ambiguities in the 1994 chronic fatigue syndrome research case definition and recommendations for resolution. *BMC Health*

Services Research, 3, 25.
Riadore, JE (1843) *Treatise on Irritation of the Spinal Nerves as the Source of Nervousness, Indigestion etc. and on the Modifying Influence of Temperament and Habits of Man over Diseases.* London: J Churchill.
Richardson, BW (1879) *Diseases of Modern Life.* London: Macmillan.
Rossetti, C (1904) *The Poetical Works of Christina Rossetti. With Memoir and Notes &c by William Michael Rossetti.* London: Macmillan.
Tennyson, A Lord (1878) *The Poetical Works of Alfred Tennyson.* London: Kegan Paul.
Savage, G (1911) Lecture on neurasthenia and mental disorders. *Medical Magazine, 20,* 620–30.
Savill, TD (1906) *Clinical Lectures on Neurasthenia* (3rd edn). London: Henry J Glaisher.
Shepherd, C (1999) *Living with ME: The chronic/post-viral syndrome.* London: Vermilion.
Shorter, E (1992) *From Paralysis to Fatigue.* New York: The Free Press.
Showalter, E (1987) *The Female Malady. Women, madness, and English culture 1830–1980.* London: Virago.
Showalter, E (1997) *Hysteries.* London: Picador.
Sinclair, J (1818) *Code of Health and Longevity or, a General View of the Rules and Principles Calculated for the Preservation of Health and the Attainment of Long Life* (4th edn). London: Henry J Glaisher.
Sontag, S (1983) *Illness as Metaphor, and Aids and its Metaphors.* Harmondsworth: Penguin.
Spencer, H (1899) *Principles of Psychology.* London: Williams & Norgate.
Spencer, H (1904) *An Autobiography* (2 Vols). London: Williams & Norgate.
Swinburne, AC (1884) *Poems and Ballads.* London: Chatto & Windus.
Swinburne, AC (1904) *The Poems of Algernon Charles Swinburne,* Vol IV. London: Chatto & Windus.
Tennyson, A (1878) *The Poetical Works of Alfred Tennyson* (Vol 1: 28). London: Kegan Paul.
Thomson, JA (1906) *Herbert Spencer.* London: JM Dent.
Wessely, S (1991) Neurasthenia and fatigue syndromes. In G Berrios & H Freeman *150 Years of British Psychiatry* (Chapter 20). London: Royal College of Psychiatrists.
Wessely, S, Hotopf, M & Sharpe, M (1998) *Chronic Fatigue and its Syndromes.* Oxford: Oxford University Press.

CHAPTER 10

ARTAUD'S MADNESS
THE ABSENCE OF WORK?

PATRICK CALLAGHAN

INTRODUCTION

This chapter is in three parts. In part one, I will introduce Antonin Artaud, and his life and work. In part two, I will examine the nature and classification of madness, drawing insights from history, the arts and humanities and social and medical sciences. In part three, I will interrogate conceptual and empirical work that enlightens us as to whether, in general, madness is the absence of work, and in particular, as Foucault has claimed, that Artaud's madness could have resulted from the absence of his work (of art).

THE LIFE AND WORK OF ANTONIN ARTAUD

Antonin Artaud was born in 1896 in Marseille, France to a French father and a Greek mother. He was a playwright, mostly adapting the work of others, usually with limited success, a theatre director, notably at the Alfred Jarry Theatre in Paris; an actor, best known for the role of the Abbot in Dreyer's classic film *The Passion of Joan of Arc*; a poet; and theatrical essayist. The latter two aspects of his work have perhaps gained him his reputation and influence with succeeding generations.

At the age of five, in 1901, it is said he suffered from meningitis. In *Antonin Artaud: The Man and His Work*, Esslin (1976), however, questions the accuracy of this diagnosis on the basis that this term was used at the turn of the twentieth century to describe various fevers and infections. The uncertainty over the diagnosis seems unlikely given that the causative agent, Neisseria meningitidis (the meningococcus), was identified in 1887, although symptoms redolent of the disease were reported much earlier (World Health Organisation, 2003). According to Esslin, Artaud himself alluded to headaches and facial cramps when aged between six and eight years. In *The Dramatic Concepts of Antonin Artaud*, Eric Sellin (1975) suggests that it was not until Artaud was 19 that he first showed signs of physical pains, but he attributes these to a side effect of mental anguish. The mental disturbances to which Sellin makes reference were to plague Artaud for the rest of his life, and resulted in frequent stays in sanatoria and mental institutions; he was to die of cancer in the sanatorium at Ivry in 1948, aged fifty-two.

When he was fourteen, Artaud, with some friends, founded a magazine in which they published a collection of poems. Artaud used a pseudonym, Louis des Attides and Sellin likens his style to that of Baudelaire and Edgar Allan Poe. In his twenties, Artaud became part of the group of artists, writers, and cultural commentators in Paris led by Andre Breton who called themselves the surrealists. He apparently wrote one-third of the surrealist manifesto, through which the group expressed their ideas. However, his flirtation with the surrealists did not last long; he was expelled for his refusal to denounce theatre as a bourgeois pursuit and for refusing to join the Communist Party.

Artaud is renowned for creating the 'Theatre of Cruelty'. In Artaud's view, theatre should be a dramatic experience that can effect change in the world. It must work with the emotions and soul of the audience and attack the audience's senses so that they may confront themselves. The Theatre of Cruelty is a method designed to use symbols of the grotesque, the ugly and pain to confront the audience's emotions. This method, described in arguably his best-known work, *The Theatre and Its Double* (1964/1993), influenced the work of playwrights Samuel Beckett and Jean Genet, director Peter Brook—at the Theatre de Bouffe Nord in Paris, Brook stages plays in a manner Artaud visualised—and the singer Jim Morrison. The Mötley Crüe's album, *Theatre of Pain*, seems to extend Artaud's ideas into a musical form. In *Madness and Civilisation,* Michel Foucault (1971) draws upon the life and work of Artaud to illustrate his postmodern views of madness.

To Sellin, Artaud's was an ironic life. For example, when in 1923 he sought publication of his poems in the French literary magazine *La Nouvelle Revue Française*, its then editor Jacques Rivière expressed little interest in the work due to its poor quality. However, Rivière was so impressed by the letters that accompanied the poems that he offered to meet Artaud, and in 1924 he published this correspondence. This irony permeated much of Artaud's life.

Like many artists, Artaud's madness seemed central to his life and work. It came as no surprise, when researching *Madness and Civilisation,* that Foucault should reference Artaud. In Foucault's view, Artaud's madness resulted from the absence of (his work of) art. In part three of this chapter, I shall return to Foucault's position on Artaud, but first, I will examine the nature and classification of madness.

SOME THOUGHTS ON THE NATURE OF MADNESS[1]

Antonin Artaud spent many years in various psychiatric hospitals, most notably at the Rodez Asylum. In his correspondence with Jacques Rivière, Artaud refers to his mental distress; *a dreadful illness of the mind,* whose origins he attributed to *the judgement of others*. There remained throughout his life episodes of what today might be classed as mental illness. Before I proceed to interrogate Foucault's arguments as to the nature of the madness Artaud experienced, I want first to examine the nature of madness.

---

1. The term 'madness' is used here to refer to any form of mental distress for which this term is but one; it is also the term Foucault uses when discussing Artaud's experiences.

Madness is a term that is universally used. It has many connotations, not all of which are seen as derogatory. The phrase, '"you don't have to be mad to work here, but it helps", suggests a light-hearted view' (BBC, 2007). Madness could also be 'mental illness: insanity, characterized by wild frenzy, mania' (*Shorter Oxford English Dictionary*, 2002, Vol 1: 1664); or denote an intense enthusiasm or fervour: to be mad, as in keen, such as when Dinah Shore sings about being *Mad About the Boy!* Citing Pascal, Foucault refers to all men being mad; the absence of madness is viewed as another form of madness in Foucault's view (Foucault, 1971). In the *Diary of a Writer*, Dostoevsky (1876/1966) writes that our own sanity is not established by the confinement of our neighbours (Artaud's judgement of others). In Hegel's view, madness is an inherent part of nature and is necessary in restoring harmony to the soul, and without madness this is not possible (Greene, 1972). The healing properties of madness are further illustrated by Hillman (1975). In *Re-visioning Psychology*, the author sees in madness the expression of the soul, not as a sickness to be remedied. (Medical) treatments fall short as a result of the medical professions' failure to recognise this view.

Various labels have been used to describe what in this paper I refer to as 'madness': mental illness, mental disorder, problems in living, abnormal psychology, psychopathology, delirium, mental sickness, psychiatric illness and social constructions of unwanted distress or phenomena. The terms most commonly used in 'official' classification manuals (e.g. *Diagnostic and Statistical Manual of Mental Disorders* (*DSM*); *International Classification of Diseases ICD-10*) are Mental Disorders and Mental and Behavioural Disorders.

The use of these terms has much to do with the fact that the care of people with mental illness has, since the eighteenth century, fallen into the hands of physicians, psychiatrists, and to a lesser extent, psychologists. These terms have little to do with a scientific explanation of the nature of madness. However, the terminology is not just a matter of semantics, the terms used by people to refer to mental illness may tells us something about the particular perspective they are adopting.

The nature of madness has been debated for centuries. From Ancient Greece (see Simon, 1978) to the present day (see Parker et al., 1995; Bentall, 2003) lay people, poets, historians, writers, psychologists, psychiatrists, nurses, sociologists, politicians and philosophers have offered differing views on madness. When one examines the statements made by people to describe madness or mental health the only conclusion worth drawing is that like beauty, madness lies in the eye of the beholder! Consider some examples:

> Mental health consists of the ability to live ... happily, productively, without being a nuisance. (Wootton, cited by Clare, 1980: 15)

> [Mental health] is the ability to maintain an even temper, an alert intelligence, socially considerate behaviour and a happy disposition. (Ibid)

> A disturbance of psychological function. (Lewis, cited in Clare, 1980: 21)

> The distraction of our mind is the result of our blind surrender to our desires, our incapacity to control or moderate our passions. (Sauvages, cited in Foucault, 1971: 85)

> Madness is no more than the derangement of the imagination. (Foucault, 1971: 93)

> A disorder exists when the failure of a person's internal mechanisms to perform the functions as designed by nature impinges harmfully on the person's well-being as defined by social values. (Wakefield, cited in Alloy, Acocella, & Bootzin, , 1996: 7)

Foucault (1971: 29–31) identifies four forms of madness: (1) Madness by romantic identification—e.g. Cervantes' Don Quixote acting out imaginary chivalry; (2) Madness of vain presumption—e.g. in Wilde's *The Picture of Dorian Gray*; (3) Madness of just punishment—King Lear, for example; and, (4) Madness of desperate passion—commonly depicted in opera, e.g. Lucia di Lammermoor, Carmen, or in Shakespeare's character, Ophelia.

Trying to define or describe madness invariably leads to attempts to distinguish normal from abnormal. According to Alloy et al (1996: 4), abnormal behaviour involves the following criteria: norm violation, statistical rarity, personal discomfort, maladaptive behaviour, deviation from the ideal, or, a combination of any or all of these.

With the differing views of what madness or health is or is not in mind, Alloy et al (1996: 7) suggest that the following categories are indicative of mental disorder across cultures:

1. Behaviour that is harmful to the self or others without serving the interests of the self. (According to Tseng et al (1995) this idea would be less relevant to some societies such as the Chinese who believe more in serving the interest of others (society), before self.)
2. Poor reality contact—for example, beliefs that most people do not hold, or sensory perceptions of things that most people do not perceive.
3. Emotional reactions inappropriate to the person's situation.
4. Erratic behaviour—that is, behaviour that shifts unpredictably.

Madness is also defined in terms of statistical norms: uncommon, extreme and infrequent behaviour; social norms: behaviour deviating from what society accepts as normal at that time; and thoughts and feelings of distress such as despair, worthlessness or hopelessness.

The above examples attempt to describe madness and mental health. There are also several perspectives that seek to explain the causes of madness.

PERSPECTIVES ON MADNESS

The *lay perspective* refers to the terms used by non-professional people. Most cultures have an opinion on those who seem to be sad, frightened, or incoherent in their behaviour (Pilgrim & Rogers, 1993). The words used to express such people and/or behaviour will obviously differ across cultures. Nevertheless, all cultures will have a lexicon to identify behaviours that seem out of keeping with that culture's norms. Often the words will refer to aspects of the person's behaviour as it affects him or her (e.g. 'that person is disturbed') or the effect of the behaviour on others (e.g. 'that person is disturbing').

The *supernatural perspective* suggests that madness results from possession by spirits or devils, 'God's revenge', 'the movement of the stars', 'the operation of evil'. This was the predominant perspective in medieval societies. As a result of such views people (mostly women) who exhibited such behaviour were often tried as witches, their treatment/punishment being death by burning.

The *medical perspective* emerged primarily in the so-called age of enlightenment (*c.* eighteenth century) although it has its roots in Ancient Greece, notably in the work of Hippocrates. Mental illness, according to this perspective, is biologically caused and results from an imbalance of bodily substances, genetic predisposition or physical trauma.

The *psychological perspectives*, which, in contrast to medical approaches, attribute madness to faulty processing in the person's interaction with his or her environment. There are many competing psychological approaches—the most widely referred to are psychodynamic, behavioural, cognitive, humanistic-existential, interpersonal and socio-cultural.

The *postmodern perspective* of madness may be traced to the work of Foucault. This perspective locates madness as a pernicious label constructed by medical practitioners through whom society gives responsibility to deal with unorthodox behaviour that it cannot, or will not, face. The effect of labelling someone as mad is to dehumanise, disenfranchise and disempower them, in other words set them apart from society's version of 'normality'.

A number of other perspectives emerged in the passage of time—the moral perspective, the familial perspective, the organic perspective. These have either gone out of fashion (the moral) or been subsumed under other perspectives (familial under psychological, organic under medical). The above perspectives seek to explain the nature, or causes of madness, they tell us little about what madness is.

CLASSIFYING MADNESS

The differences in defining and describing madness led to a concerted effort by psychiatrists to develop classification systems that would be relevant for use across cultures and which could be used by clinicians to detect, diagnose and treat it. The two classification systems used are the *Diagnostic and Statistical Manual of Mental Disorders,* now in its fourth edition, (*DSM-IV-TR*) published by the American Psychiatric

Table 1. A comparison of different perspectives of madness

Criterion	Psychosocial	Biomedical
Causes of illness	Behaviour, beliefs, coping, stress, poverty, socio-economic inequalities	Viruses, bacteria, lesions
Responsibility for illness	Individual and social, political, economic and environmental forces	External forces causing internal changes
Treatment of illness	Holistically: Changes in beliefs, behaviour, and coping styles, reduce or eradicate inequalities	Medication
Responsibility for treatment	The person, family unit, community, support networks	The doctor and other agencies in collaboration with the user
Relationship between mental health and illness	Both exist on a continuum: degrees of health–illness	Dichotomous: the person is either healthy or ill
Relationship between mind and body	Mind and body inter-dependent	Mind and body function independently of one another
Role in health and illness	Psychosocial factors contribute to mental health status	Illness has psychosocial consequences, not psychosocial causes

Association in 2004 and the *International Classification of Mental and Behavioural Disorders*, now in its tenth revision (*ICD-10*), published by the World Health Organisation in 1992.

These classification systems have gone some way to redress some of the chaos that existed in previous attempts to classify madness in a manner that was satisfactory, valid, and had cross-cultural relevance. However, they have been criticised for their 'failure to represent the diversity of human experiences of distress' (Parker et al, 1995: 37). Parker et al also cite criticisms of the *DSM* and *ICD-10* on the grounds that they reflect commercial interests, are individualistic, reflect dominant conceptions of the Western self, are social constructions, and are empirically invalid. They represent truth, but only by the consensus agreement (Bentall, 2003). They also argue that these systems fail to account for the influences of race, identity, gender, class, and social power in people's experiences of distress. In short, Parker et al argue that attempts to classify madness are futile, unhelpful, and contribute little to alleviating people's distress. Newton (1988: 19) argues, however, that classification systems help determine the ill from the moderately or mildly ill. The absence of such systems, she continues, would hamper our ability to plan services, evaluate the success of treatment and rehabilitation, or to assess the effectiveness of preventive strategies.

MADNESS AND THE ABSENCE OF WORK

In his conclusion to *Madness and Civilisation*, Foucault (1971) suggests that madness results from the absence of a work of art, but also recognises that madness is also synonymous with this work (pp 288–9). Referring to artists such as Goya, Van Gogh and Artaud, Foucault states although these people were mad they managed to create works of art, thus the fissure between reason and madness is joined by the art. Madness is not revealed through the application of science or reason, but through the absence of a work of art:

> Artaud's madness does not slip through the fissures of a work of art; his madness is precisely the absence of the work of art. (p. 287)

The extent to which madness is the absence of work is the focus of the remaining part of this chapter. I shall start with a critique of empirical literature in which researchers investigate the relationship between work and madness.

The Greek physician Galen (c. 130–200), arguably one of the most influential figures in medical history, believed that employment, which he regarded as nature's physician, was fundamental to people's happiness. Galen's prescient views are supported by contemporary findings (Waddell & Burton, 2006). Employment is recognised as an important means through which people with mental health problems and disengaged from society can re-engage. Attaining gainful, productive and paid employment is seen as fundamental to helping people recover from incapacitating mental health problems, and is a key strand of recovery approaches (Sainsbury Centre for Mental Health (SCMH), 2007; Repper & Perkins, 2003). One reason for advocating employment in such approaches is that it confers a sense of social inclusion, i.e. people previously marginalised from society as a result of mental health problems or unemployment can become better integrated. In his report on the state of mental health services, the National Director for Mental Health in England emphasised the importance of 're-defining recovery to incorporate quality of life—a job, a decent place to live, friends and a social life' (Department of Health, 2007a).

Work also promotes social support as it invariably provides people with an enlarged social network that has the potential to enhance a person's health. Having access to a network of social contacts who provide satisfactory levels of support is instrumental to quality of life, and has also been shown to enhance mental health and well-being; the absence of social support is linked to psychiatric morbidity and premature mortality (Callaghan & Morrissey, 1993; Lam & Rosenheck, 1999).

In his C.S. Myers lecture at the British Psychological Society's annual conference in Brighton in 1994, David Fryer from the University of Stirling quotes Marie Jahoda, an eminent social psychologist renowned for her studies on unemployment and health:

> [E]mployment makes the following categories of experience inevitable: it imposes a time structure on the waking day; it compels contacts and shared experiences with others outside the nuclear family; it demonstrates that there are goals and purposes which are beyond the scope of an individual but require a collectivity; it imposes status and social identity through the division of labour in modern employment; it enforces activity ... (Jahoda, quoted in Sterling, 1994)

Work confers status and identity. Work provides a salary and position that allows people to attain, or maintain a certain status in society. The status and identity attained from working is linked to improvements in self-esteem. Work also provides people with an identity over and above that conferred by other roles in life, such as father, mother or partner (Waddell & Burton, 2006).

Invariably work provides a means of structuring and occupying time. Most jobs involve some form of structure and regulated hours; people in work will know generally where they will be between these hours, and other activity, such as leisure, is usually organised outside these times. For most people, this structured and regulated time will account for almost half of their life expectancy. Work can instil a sense of personal achievement as it often provides opportunities to learn and master a craft or skill, opportunities that may not otherwise be available. Often the skills people learn at work may be applied more widely outside the work place. This reinforces the sense of achievement and also enhances opportunities for further financial reward.

Work may reduce relative and absolute poverty as it provides a means through which people can achieve shelter, a fundamental human need. Work also allows access to goods and services which often impact positively on people's quality of life and well-being, such as holidays.

Finally, work promotes recovery, leads to better health, buffers people against the harmful effects of long-term sickness absence, improves quality of life and well-being, and reduces social exclusion and poverty (Waddell & Burton, 2006).

In summary, there is evidence that work is generally good for our health and well-being. However, there are caveats: not all work confers the benefits reported above; jobs seen as menial are less likely to provide such benefits. There may be more advantages to being unemployed for some people.

In *Nickel and Dimed*, the American author Barbara Ehrenreich (2002) reports her experience of an experiment of spending a year working in a variety of jobs that paid below the national minimum wage in the USA. The account of her own experiences, and those of the people she encountered in this year, tell of widespread exploitation, abuse, harm and degradation suffered by many employees. Although Ehrenreich was well educated, was in good health, had her own car and enough money to pay her rent for at least a month, Ehrenreich found it necessary to do two jobs, often working seven days per week. Despite these resources, she still found herself on the brink of needing to live in a hostel for homeless people.

Likewise, in *Fast Food Nation*, Eric Schlosser (2002) recounts a similar tale from the perspective of people working in industries that supply the ingredients for the food people buy in so-called fast food restaurants. These experiences are being shared by an increasing number of people worldwide; being employed does not buffer everyone from the effects of poverty (United Nations, 2000; Sachs, 2005). The European Union (EU) notes that:

> While good mental health increases work capacity and productivity, poor working conditions including the intimidation by colleagues lead to poor mental health, sick leave and increased costs; up to 28% of employees in Europe report stress at work. (EU, 2005: 9)

Having considered the effects of work on mental health and well-being, I shall now examine what happens in the absence of work, with particular reference to the evidence linking madness to the absence of work.

Madness often destroys people's creativity and impairs their ability to work. Approximately 20% of work absences in the United Kingdom are due to mental health problems. Unemployment among people with mental health problems is around 87% and is linked to depression, parasuicide, and in some cases suicide itself. For most people, unemployment is a significantly distressing life event and may even decrease life expectancy (Ezzy, 1993; Owen & Watson, 1995; Murphy & Athanasou, 1999; Welch, 2001; McLean et al., 2005; Woolston, 2006).

For the purposes of trying to ascertain whether madness is the absence of work I have chosen as an operational definition of madness any experience that leads to incapacitating distress that may threaten life, quality of life, mental health and well-being and impede a person's ability to attend to everyday activities that also bring solace.

There is a strong relationship between unemployment and psychopathology (McLean et al, 2005). For some, unemployment is pathogenic (Shortt, 1996). Unemployment may be linked to increases in health-related behaviours like alcohol use, but the evidence is inconclusive. There is evidence of a link between unemployment and suicide, although in the United Kingdom (UK) there is stronger evidence that unemployment is linked to attempted suicide (McLean et al, 2005); however, previous suicide attempts are a strong predictor of future suicide (DH, 2007b).

When using common measures of mental health, such as the General Health Questionnaire (GHQ), studies show strong associations between unemployment and increased prevalence of mental disorders such as depression, anxiety, as well as decreases in life satisfaction, self-esteem, and hopelessness (McLean et al, 2005; Warr, 2002). In its Green Paper on Mental Health, the EU (2005) shows that unemployment can lower self-esteem and lead to depression.

While the absence of work is linked to 'madness' a cautionary note is sounded. Empirical studies linking the absence of work to mental ill health fail to demonstrate a causal link and do not consider that psychological attributes such as locus of control, self-efficacy and resilience may mitigate the adverse effects of unemployment. Also, there are other mitigating factors such as gender, age, ethnicity, socio-economic status, financial anxiety, education level and pre-unemployment status, and the state of the economy that are often overlooked. People who choose to leave their jobs seldom suffer the same consequences as those who are made redundant (Woolston, 2006).

Of course there is a long history and prolific literature linking madness and creativity: the work of Sylvia Plath, Strindberg, Emily Dickinson, Tennessee Williams, Eugene O'Neill, William Faulkner, Van Gogh, and Munch, for example. Taking the opposite view that madness is the absence of work, Jeremy Reed's (1989) analysis of the work of poets such as Rilke, Baudelaire, Rimbaud, John Clare and Gerard Manley Hopkins suggests that the exceptional and compelling gift of poetry exerts a high price; in Reed's view, madness is that price.

In *Madness and Creativity: New Findings and Old Stereotypes*, Rothenberg (1994) takes a contrary view. Rothenburg argues that the best works of so-called mad figures occurred during bouts of rationality, sanity and remission. This brings us back to Artaud.

Artaud's life was characterised by bouts of despair, insanity and incapacitating distress, but he also appeared to enjoy periods of great lucidity and clarity of mind. This is evident in several works. In his lengthy correspondence with Jacques Rivière, he articulated lucidly the ideas of how he constructed the poems that inspired the correspondence. Rivière was impressed by Artaud's prowess in literary criticism, but remained unimpressed by the poems themselves. For Rivière, Artaud demonstrated extraordinary insight into his own condition of mind, whilst recognising the quality of his critiques of his own literary efforts, Rivière, nevertheless contrasted this with the poems themselves, which he considered vague and shapeless. At time of the correspondence, Artaud refers to the illness of his mind—a horrible sickness; the poems he sent, and the correspondence that accompanied them were wreckage that he rescued from a mental void. Whereas the madness to which Artaud appears to be alluding in this correspondence may have impeded his poetry, it appears not to have inhibited his literary skill, at least in the judgement of others, in this case Rivière, another irony.

The Theatre and Its Double (1964/1993) outlines Artaud's views on the theatre in general, and his ideas for a Theatre of Cruelty in particular, and is arguably his most influential work. The text is an illustration of the ironies and contradictions of Artaud's life; an influential treatise on theatre; a seeming inability to produce a play of note—the absence of work.

On one hand, Artaud presents highly original ideas that he expresses with fluency, on the other, moments of incomprehensible technicality. In a letter to Jean Paulhan in 1936, Artaud refers to many doubles (i.e. reflections of the the theatre in life, and vice versa) of the theatre: metaphysics, plague and cruelty, conditions that could easily sum up his own life. So it is not surprising to find in these conditions a juxtaposition for his ideas on theatre.

Madness bedevilled Artaud for most of his adult life, and this seems to have encumbered his work. Nowhere is this better illustrated than in the programme he devised for French radio, shortly before his death, *To Have Done with the Judgement of God*. This programme was commissioned as part of a series *Voices of Poets* (Esslin, 1976). Artaud does not so much recite the poems, as scream the words in cries of anguish, torment and inarticulacy. There can be little doubt of the madness that lies behind these utterances. According to Esslin (1976), they must go beyond madness, but he is unable to state exactly what these utterances represent, other than to suggest that if they were mere madness, Artaud's posthumous reputation would be less than it is.

Like King Lear's catharsis in the storm, Artaud's laments as represented in *To Have Done with the Judgement of God* acted as a catalyst for a different way of seeing for future artists. In this way, Esslin likens the enduring impact of Artaud's work on successive generations to that of Che Guevara, i.e. as an enduring symbol of a particular genre. Unlike, Guevara, however, Artaud's legacy is appreciated by a somewhat esoteric group. Artaud's madness therefore both fuelled and stalled his oeuvre.

Madness, therefore, is the absence of work, but also its catalyst. Madness can be both a curse and a blessing. For in madness lies the possibility of enlightenment and renewal. Through madness Lear was able to comprehend the machinations of others. Madness gave Hamlet time to reflect, asylum from the torment of his grief. Through the fug of his madness, Artaud was able to articulate a vision of the possibilities of how we may experience great Art, and how others might realize it on our behalf.

REFERENCES

Alloy, LB, Acocella, J & Bootzin, RR (1996) *Abnormal Psychology: Current perspectives* (7th edn). New York: McGraw-Hill.

American Psychiatric Association (2004) *The Diagnostic and Statistical Manual of Mental Disorders* (4th edn, Text Revision). Washington, DC: American Psychiatric Association.

Artaud, A (1964/1993) *The Theatre and Its Double*. London: Calder.

Artaud, A (1970) *Antonin Artaud: Collected Works* (Vols 1–4). London: Calder.

Artaud, A (1988) *Selected Writings*. Berkeley, CA/Los Angeles, CA: University of California Press.

Bentall, R (2003) *Madness Explained*. London: Penguin/Allen Lane.

British Broadcasting Corporation (2002) Madness. Accessed 10th January 2008 at <www.bbc.co.uk/dna/h2g2/A694604>.

Callaghan, P & Morrissey, J (1993) Social support and health: A review. *Journal of Advanced Nursing, 18,* 203–10.

Clare, A (1980) *Psychiatry in Dissent: Controversial issues in thought and practice* (2nd edn). London: Tavistock.

Department of Health (2007a) *Breaking Down Barriers: Clinical case for change*. Report by Louis Appleby, National Director for Mental Health. London: DH.

Department of Health, (2007b) *Best Practice in Managing Risk*. London: DH.

Dostoevsky, FM (1966) *Diary of a Writer* (DV Grishin, Trans). Melbourne: University of Melbourne.
Ehrenreich, B (2002) *Nickel and Dimed: Undercover in low-wage America*. London: Granta.
Esslin, M (1976) *Antonin Artaud: The man and his work*. London: Calder.
European Union (2005) *Green Paper on Mental Health*. Brussels: EU.
Ezzy, D (1993) Unemployment and mental health: a critical review. *Social Science and Medicine*, 37 (1), 41–52.
Foucault, M (1971) *Madness and Civilisation: A history of insanity in the age of reason*. London: Routledge.
Greene, M (1972) *Hegel on the Soul*. The Hague: Nijhoff.
Hillman, J (1975) *Re-visioning Psychology*. London: Harper & Row.
Lam, JA & Rosenheck, R (1999) Social support and service use among homeless persons with serious mental illness. *International Journal of Social Psychiatry*, 45 (1), 13–18.
McLean, C, Camona, C, Francis, S, Wohlgemuth, C & Mulvivhill, C (2005) *Worklessness and Health: What do we know about the causal relationship?* (1st edn). London: Health Development Agency. Accessed 14th October 2007 at <www.hda.nhs.uk/evidence>.
Murphy, GC & Athanasou, JA (1999) The effects of unemployment on mental health. *Journal of Occupational and Organisational Psychology*, 72, 83–99.
Newton, J (1988) *Preventing Mental Illness*. London: Routledge.
Owen, K & Watson, N (1995) Unemployment and mental health. *Journal of Psychiatric and Mental Health Nursing*, 2, 63–71.
Parker, I, Geogarca, E, Harper, D, McLaughlin, T & Stowell-Smith, M (1995) *Deconstructing Psychopathology*. London: Sage.
Pilgrim, D & Rogers, A (1993) *A Sociology of Mental Health and Illness*. Buckingham: Open University Press.
Reed, J (1989) *Madness: The price of poetry*. London: Peter Owen.
Repper, J & Perkins, R (2003) *Social Inclusion and Recovery*. Edinburgh: Baillière Tindall.
Rothenburg, A (1994) *Madness and Creativity: New findings and old stereotypes*. Baltimore, MD: John Hopkins University Press.
Sachs, J (2005) *The End of Poverty*. New York: United Nations.
Sainsbury Centre for Mental Health (2007) *Mental Health and Employment*. Briefing Paper 33. London: Sainsbury Centre for Mental Health.
Schlosser, E (2002) *Fast Food Nation: What the all-American meal is doing to the world*. London: Penguin.
Sellin, E (1975) *The Dramatic Concepts of Antonin Artaud*. Chicago: Chicago University Press.
Shorter Oxford English Dictionary. (2002) (5th edn). Oxford: Oxford University Press.
Shortt, SED (1996) Is unemployment pathogenic? A review of current concepts with lessons for policy planners. *International Journal of Health Services*, 26 (3), 569–89.
Simon, B (1978) *Mind and Madness in Ancient Greece: The classical roots of modern psychiatry*. Ithaca, NY/London: Cornell University Press.
Sterling, D (1994) C.S. Myers lecture at the British Psychological Society's annual conference in Brighton. Accessed 21st May 2007 at <http://www.jobsletter.org.nz/jbl02410.htm>.
Tseng, WS, Lin, TY & Eng, KY (1995) Chinese societies and mental health. In WS Tseng et al (Eds) *Chinese Societies and Mental Health* (pp 3–18). Hong Kong: Oxford University Press.
United Nations (2000) *Overcoming Human Poverty*. New York, United Nations. Accessed 6th February 2008 at <www.undp.org/povertyreport>.

Waddell, G & Burton, AK (2006) *Is Work Good for Your Health and Well-Being?* London: The Stationery Office.

Warr, P (2002) *The Psychology of Work* (5th edn). London: Penguin.

Welch, S (2001) A review of the literature on the epidemiology of parasuicide in the general population. *Psychiatric Services, 52* (3), 368–75.

Woolston, C (2006) *Why Unemployment is Bad for Your Health.* Accessed 16th July 2008 at <http://ahealthyme.com/topic/unemployment>.

World Health Organisation (1992) *The ICD-10 Classification of Mental and Behavioural Disorders: Clinical descriptions and diagnostic guidelines.* Geneva: WHO.

World Health Organisation (2003) *Meningococcal Meningitis.* Fact Sheet 141. Geneva: WHO.

Chapter 11

A PHENOMENOLOGICAL ENCOUNTER
PRELUDE TO A MENTAL HEALTH ASSESSMENT IN A MAGISTRATE'S CELLS

Dave R. Wilson

This paper describes the context and processes involved in providing mental health support to a large magistrates' court. More specifically, the paper seeks to explore how eye contact is used as a means of establishing 'a relationship' with an unknown Other, assessing the Other's potential risk to Self, and how that fleeting, pre-verbal momentary experience gives rise to a range of perceptual meanings and value weightings for the two people involved.

To this end, the paper will focus on the few seconds when, with the decision made to assess a specific individual, that individual is escorted from the cells, along a corridor, and into the space that gives access to the interview rooms. The room designated for use by the Mental Health Officer (MHO) is ten standard paces away from the point where the prospective assessee and assessor first have the opportunity to physically set eyes on one another.

The kind of relational events that may or may not occur, in the One's traversing of that silent space and across those ten paces (toward the Other), forms the substance of this paper.

This paper assumes that:

> [W]ithout any special reflection we attribute to everyone else our own constitution and therefore our own consciousness as well, and that this identification is a sine qua non of our understanding. (Freud, cited by Strachey, in Nagel, 1995: 18)

THE CONTEXT

There is a very literal descent involved in moving from the public areas of the magistrates' court to the cellblock area. One has to take the elevator down and away from a world of carpeted offices with windows, standing plants, water dispensers, and people in very expensive suits.

After passing through several locked doors and voided spaces (i.e. past the outer police cordon and into a cellblock area staffed by a private security firm), one arrives at a place with no windows or natural light of any kind, and a complete absence of standing plants or the kind of bric-à-brac one might usually associate with a 'human working environment'. An area is given over to interview rooms and cubicles, and beyond these spaces, deeper inside the building, are the cells themselves.

The interview rooms are painted an all-over pastel green. The furniture in each of the interview rooms consists of a bolted-down table with two bolted-down chairs (one on either side of the table). The rooms are each the size of an average 'twelve persons standing' elevator, and just as visually uninteresting—unless reports of feelings of claustrophobia from previously non-claustrophobic persons counts as 'interesting'. A large blue 'panic button' is situated close to the door inside each room. This button, if depressed, would result in large numbers of cell staff appearing at the door very quickly. The fact that, over ten years, no member of the Court Assessment Team (i.e. a team of forensic community psychiatric nurses who act as the MHO on a rotational basis) has ever had to press that button is, the author contests, a tribute to the pre-assessment decision-making skills of the individual MHOs, the good lines of communication that exist between the Court Assessment Team members and the cell staff (this includes valuing the experience and 'lay wisdom' of the cell staff), and the communication and interpersonal skills of individual MHOs once locked in the interview room with the detained Other for the duration of the assessment, or until the Other is summoned by the magistrate.

The fact that the magistrate can summon the detained individual to court at any moment complicates the whole assessment process. For, if one accepts that assessing someone in such circumstances is a difficult enough task without any time constraints, then the inclusion of an 'uncertainty factor', with regard to how much time the MHO has to complete the task, necessarily has consequences within the interaction itself. For instance, even with a robust and reliable (i.e. user-friendly and evidence-based) assessment instrument, an amenable and articulate Other, and the appropriate level of communication and interpersonal skills on the part of the MHO, the uncertainty about how much or how little time the MHO has to conduct the assessment often results in a pressure to forego many of the social conventions or 'getting to know you' scenarios which, in other circumstances, could nurture trust and rapport, as well as enhancing the quality of information obtained. For instance, 'ordinary chat' or phatic communication, as 'language used in free, aimless, social intercourse' (Burnard, 2003: 678, quoting Malinowski, 1922), wherein the conversation is more important than the subject, is, in such circumstances, an early casualty. Hence, the very urgency of the situation tends to result in a formalising of an interaction that, ideally, needs less rather than more formality built into its scene-setting and scripting.

So, it is against this background that the MHO is suddenly 'introduced' to, usually, an 'unknown Other', while The Other is faced with, often, the 'threat' of an unknown 'professional Other' (e.g. a 'nutter nurse' who they may think could 'nut me off' [i.e. under a Section of the Mental Health Act, 1983]), with neither knowing the duration of the encounter, nor what the outcome of the encounter and assessment might entail.

TENARAY: A MAN UNTO HIMSELF

For the purposes of this paper, a hypothetical alleged offender, named Tenaray (from an old African term meaning 'where there is nothing', or, in this case, no specific individual), will be employed to aid clarity by providing specific examples of types of eye contact and behaviour. Tenaray has been charged with stealing brie and grape sandwiches from a famous high-street store—the fourth such offence, of the same type of sandwiches, from the same store, at the same time of day, and with the same consequences (i.e. arrest and bail), in the last four days.

As Tenaray and his Escort turn the corner from the cells and into the author's view, the 'I-as-MHO' (i.e. the professional 'character' created to meet the needs of the circumstances and the task in hand) adopts a well-practiced stance in the doorframe of the MHO's assessment room. Eye contact has not yet been engaged, but the MHO is already actively observing and perceiving.

SETTING THE SCENE, THE OBSERVING EYE, AND THE POWER OF A DOORFRAME

> Staff face-to-face with a relatively unknown patient have only one source of information readily available with which to make an assessment of violence risk; the verbal and non-verbal behaviour of the patient, i.e. what the patient is saying and doing at a particular moment. (Whittington & Patterson, 1996: 48)

In the context of a magistrate's cells environment, the author would add a caveat to Whittington and Patterson's (1996) statement. This, to the effect that one also needs to gather data about what Tenaray *isn't* saying and *isn't* doing at a particular moment, as well as from one moment to the next, within the 'sizing-up of one another', or, less brutally, perhaps, within the dual process of gauging the Other's risk to Self. For the earliest instants of each gaze will tend, particularly in the prevailing circumstances, to rouse the sympathetic nervous systems of the protagonists, and the 'fight-or-flight' impulse has to be overcome—or negotiated around—before each individual's functional levels of 'stranger anxiety' begin to shape and determine the more communicative and qualitative eye-to-eye interactions or encounters.

> We look at a person and immediately a certain impression of his character forms itself in us. A glance ... [is] sufficient to tell us a story about a highly complex matter ... we also know that this process, though often imperfect [and] perhaps informed by our idols [see below], is also at times extraordinarily sensitive. (Asch, cited in Henle, 1961)

These 'first impressions' are vitally important, as they will set the foundations for the success or failure of the imminent verbal encounter. According to Gladwell (2005), such moments involve, not just one's conscious observational skills, but the unbidden and almost instantaneous harvesting of faint impressions and conclusions that our 'adaptive unconscious' brings to our attention in what he terms a process of 'thin-slicing' (i.e. a time-limited process whereby a thin slice of an interaction [e.g. three seconds from a video recording of a conversation or activity] can, he argues, generate decisions about a person that are just as accurate, or, perhaps, more accurate than, say, an hour-long interview). Kihlstrom (1996) provides an excellent example of the Adaptive Unconscious at work, though Kihlstrom gives the thin-slicing process the title of 'The Judas Eye'. The Judas Eye was, during the Prohibition-era in America, 'the peephole' (in entrance doors to speakeasies) 'through which a bouncer could determine who could be admitted, a determination that required that the person be identified'. Such an 'identification' would often be as much about the judgement the bouncer made, about the content of his Perception (i.e. 'does he look alright?' 'does he look like a cop?'), as it was by recognition of someone from a previous visit, or any written proofs of identification. In short, Kihlstrom (1996) suggests that there is a level of perception, of recognition, that registers information 'below [conscious] awareness in the perceptual-cognitive system' (p. 24). While provisionally accepting Kihlstrom's view, the MHO also has to accept that, what some might dismiss as a form of 'intuition', needs to be closely monitored with regard to the extent to which The Judas Eye might influence other perceptions (see 'The Secreting-away of "Idols"', below).

Indeed, being aware of and fully understanding the roots of impressions represented to the MHO by so-called 'objective observation' and the Adaptive Unconscious/Judas Eye (hereafter, The Judas Eye), or some combination of both, and being able to distinguish the one form of perceiving from the other, requires considerable self-knowledge and skill on the part of the MHO.

Also, insofar as The One individual is being brought into contact with The Other precisely because of a perceived instability, or risk, relating to The One (i.e. Tenaray), makes of every instant, every 'discreet sequence' of time, an opportunity for both parties to undertake a significant thin-slicing of the Other. Indeed, the author hopes to demonstrate that the perceptions-meanings acquired in the bracketed/thin-sliced periods of time between the author's hearing (and smelling) Tenaray, and our first verbal exchange, are not only important in themselves, in terms of identifying potential risk factors (on both sides), but that they provide the conscious and unconscious qualitative basis for the subsequent success or failure of the verbal encounter.

The perceiving-meaning of the totality (i.e. employing some combination of [experientially based] conscious and Judas Eye observations) of Tenaray's presentation is also essential in identifying and then subjectively 'rating' a huge range of non-verbal communications. Such communications are well documented (e.g. Silverman et al, 1998), but in the present context a number of basic cues or clues pertain: posture, body movements and gestures, facial expression, vocal cues (e.g. noises, grunts, groans), physical presence (e.g. clothing, gender, 'grooming'), and eye contact, or its lack. These 'observables' are then compared and contrasted with the impressionistic material that, according to Gladwell (2005) and Kihlstrom (1996), our equally skilled Adaptive Unconscious/Judas Eye is likely to have already made available to each of us.

Tenaray presents as relaxed, even confident in his movements. He is in his late twenties, is short of stature but built like a prop-forward, and he has no shoes or socks on. His clothes appear to evidence the grime of many nights spent on the streets. Indeed, the smell of stale urine had reached my nostrils long before I set eyes on Tenaray. He is engaged in what appears to be a jovial enough conversation with his escort, and has not yet looked in the direction of the MHO.

Yet, I seem to know this man. I've met this man before. I cannot find him in Memory, but the impression conveyed to me via, perhaps, a shard of memory being further informed by something out of The Judas Eye, causes a sense of growing unease. The I-as-MHO sets this feeling, this presently vague unease, aside. After all, such unease is not in keeping with the creation of what will be termed 'a tranquil receptivity'.

JUST STANDING STOOD THERE

Presenting and maintaining a relaxed, non-threatening, and seemingly unself-conscious stance, while feeling all too self-conscious and in trying to deal with one's own variable levels of 'stranger-anticipatory anxiety', demands mental discipline and a very self-aware, very skilled actor. Indeed, the total situation lends itself to a certain 'theatricality' insofar as the cell space area provides a stage, the MHO is one role, the smell of Tenaray announces a *building* of his role 'in the wings', and there will be at least one I-as-Spectator. Indeed, 'the pejorative use of the term *theatricality* as mere surface or show thus fails to take into account the more strategic use of show as an interactive trap' (Freedman, 1991)—though the idea of 'a trap' raises its own ethical issues. That said, it is worth noting that in similar situations on the selfsame stage, an overt, almost pantomime-like or theatrical obviousness, both in terms of the improvised script and actions of the actors, has actually served to give The Other actor 'permission' to *disclose* (i.e. to disclose that which otherwise might have remained hidden)—or is the disclosure a direct result of The One trapping The Other?

On a more everyday level, this not-so-fondly imagined self-regarding, self-monitoring (Ideal) Self also requires the MHO to attend to and be able to identify, in the non-verbal and verbal behaviour of The Other, any overt or obvious indicators (e.g. crying; shouting; being argumentative and demanding; aggressive gesturing or attempts to physically assault another or to hurt themselves; or signs and symptoms of psychotic experiencing) or more covert indicators (e.g. emotional-psychological distance or vacancy; the appearance of shame; seeming indifference, or arrogance in the face of current circumstances; or signs and symptoms of psychotic experiencing), that might require some subtle or less subtle shift in emphasis in the MHO's 'just standing stood there' performance.

Although terms like 'actors' and 'performance' may not be considered the best words to describe the situation or the MHO's gathering together of genuine aspects of

Self, in order, then, to meet the needs of the current circumstances, it will suffice. For, if we humans were stripped of our socially constructed actor/performance skills, one would have to wonder how first encounters, or interactions, could progress to form the basis of complex and lasting relationships.

So, depending on The Other's physical-behavioural presentation, the MHO may have to re-chisel that open, cheerful silhouette into one of an appropriate 'serious intensity', or, perhaps, a more non-committal 'tranquil receptivity'. This physical responsiveness has to be flexible enough, and replete with a continuum of chameleon-like nuances, to communicate to this Tenaray the fact that the MHO is seeking to make a connection, to communicate, via a form of non-verbal physical-mirroring-responding, that there is a recognition of The Other's subjective distress or, at the very least, his current situation.

On the odd occasion when The Other's presentation is so chaotic and ever-changing, say, from one step to the next, then there is the risk that the unsubtle or overly responsive MHO could make him/herself look ridiculous (i.e. through a physical pantomime involving multiple sculptural changes that, taken as a sequence, could be construed as 'the agitation of the insecure', an itchy infestation, or of some mental disturbance), in the eyes of The Other, The Escort, The Assessor's Ideal Self, and, even, The 'performing' I-as-MHO.

But how, I hear the reader ask, does one sculpture one's physical form into 'a tranquil receptivity'? Well, the process requires an 'artistic' (Benner, 1984; Wiedenbach, 1985), combination of individual, experientially evolved, acting/performing skills that provide an outward display, an outward 'reciprocal mirror' (i.e. insofar as the physical sculptor is also trying to respond appropriately to the Other's physical-emotional presentation), of a mood or mental state that has, as its base, a particular receptive quality. That quality is, here, consistent with what phenomenologists term, 'the phenomenal attitude' (see 'Phenomenology: Issues of Perception and Meaning', below).

In the meantime, and for the moment, the doorway to the interview room provides both a literal and a metaphorical frame for the MHO's performance. The act of standing in the frame of the door could be perceived of as carrying myriad sub-texts of meaning that The Other may or may not recognise. Given the situational context (i.e. The Other is in custody and is about to go before a magistrate charged with a criminal offence), many of these sub-texts could relate to Power and Powerlessness (e.g. who, in the environment, has power, and who hasn't). For instance, there's 'the territorial imperative' (with apologies to Ardrey, 1967)—the 'rule of Nature' wherein the creature holding, or being otherwise in control of the territory or place, is perceived to be in a position of dominance over 'the intruder'. Hence, by positioning myself in the doorframe, and effectively barring access to '*my* interview room', I-as-MHO assert my dominance, my power over, in this case, Tenaray. Such a stance is hardly conducive to my, then, attempting to manifest a 'tranquil receptivity'. This tranquil receptivity also includes the communication, via reciprocal mirroring, of a basic recognition or understanding of The Other and/or his situation. However, by standing in the doorframe, and then stepping aside to offer Tenaray entry into the interview room, a mini-barrage of, hopefully, more positive meanings, may be transmitted to him. These meanings, if received by Tenaray in the manner described, might include sub-texts like; 'here, you have a choice (i.e. to enter or not)'; 'I (the MHO), though I have choices and powers that you (Tenaray) do not currently possess, I choose not to exercise some of those choices or powers to your detriment'; or, more simply, 'please, do come in'.

Across a decade, the author can attest to having stood in that doorframe as every manner of alleged offender, from the loftiest of 'social heights' to the depths of social, physical, and mental desolation, and with any number or combination of presentations (e.g. from shame and self-loathing to indignant rage, from a form of *schadenfreudean* self-satisfaction, or 'joy in the misery of others', that emanates from one who has 'paid somebody back', to a 'traumatic numbness' or a psychopathic indifference, and from genuine fear and anxiety to active psychosis), has traversed that ten-pace space.

In the context of this cell's environment, I have found it useful, if somewhat ethically 'uncomfortable', firstly, to reinforce the actual nature of The Other's circumstances and relative powerlessness (i.e. by standing in the doorframe), and, secondly, to then appear to sunder that power by stepping aside to offer The Other entry into the interview room. I say 'appear to sunder that power' because, essentially, Tenaray's circumstances and my role as the MHO—with all the inequities that our roles imply—remain utterly unchanged. Indeed, the extent of my power over Tenaray is clearly demonstrated in the fact that I have the ability to 'set the scene'—a man stood in a doorway—while Tenaray is brought to me, more or less willingly, a stranger in an unfamiliar place, and a stranger, moreover, without a doorframe of his own.

Instead of a doorframe, Tenaray comes into the MHO's visual domain with an escort. And what, one could ask, is the power differential between Tenaray and his Escort (i.e. the person who has brought Tenaray from a cell and who will shortly be returning him to that place [or to the court] and locking him in)? This is a question that merits a paper in itself and, consequently, it is only partially addressed here. But, just as the MHO utilises the physical environment (i.e. the doorframe and my positioning within it, or to the side of it) to send The Other signals or messages, so The Other, usually unintentionally, also communicates a great deal to the MHO. This is achieved by virtue of the interpersonal dynamics that manifest themselves in the interactions—or lack of interactions—between The Other and his Escort, as they turn into the MHO's view and commence the ten paces to the interview room's doorframe. As already stated, Tenaray is engaged in a cheerful enough and, more importantly for the MHO, articulate and appropriately flowing dialogue with his escort.

It is not the customary practice for The Other and The Escort to be handcuffed to one another in the cellblock area, so their walking together, in the context that one is in the custody of the other, has the potential for some form of normalcy. For 'normalcy', read two men in close proximity, not touching one another, walking in the same direction, and each with clearly defined roles within their interaction/relationship—in short, two men in, usually, a silent dialogue of mutual conforming.

On those few occasions when The Other has been in handcuffs, or has been in handcuffs and was being escorted by four or six escorts, or was presenting in what appeared to be a florid psychotic state (e.g. 'Lilith, God will smite thee, along with these, thy devilish spawn [the Escorts]'), that silent dialogue of mutual conformity has been absent. In such circumstances, the loss of the 'mutual conformity' benchmark is invariably replaced by a considerably more complex array of dynamic interactions that the MHO must rapidly assess.

In general, though, and as I have my doorframe with which to make my power manifest, so the seemingly disempowered Tenaray can engage with his Escort, or not, and in so doing, may attempt to establish—for himself, to the Escort, and for the benefit of any observers, that neither the Escort nor anyone else has any real power over him; or that the Escort has absolute power over him; or that, whatever their relation is to one another, Tenaray has a 'face-saver' in place that overrides the Escort's real or imagined power over him.

Hence, The One may engage in light banter with The Other. If the two know one another well, their conversation may have all the appearance of two friends engaging in the kind of mundane, phatic chatter that friends often do—more especially when walking together toward the same object (i.e. task) or destination. For example:

> Tenaray (in feigned innocence): *Hey, Mick, you're a Manchester United supporter aren't you?*
> Mick/Escort (with knowing humour and with mock suspiciousness): *Yeah, ... and?*
> Tenaray (victorious): *Didn't they get well ******* beaten last night.*

Alternatively, the content of the verbal or non-verbal dialogue, or utter lack of dialogue, may be indicative of another Tenaray's shame, guilt, hatred, fear, loathing, indifference, anxiety, or insanity, or any combination of these. For example, after recognising the mortal fear in a man's eyes as he walked the ten paces—fifteen shuffling reluctant steps for him—to the interview room, I subsequently discovered that he had thought he was being brought to his own execution, that some horrendous and macabre death awaited him in the room whose doorframe I had so kindly stepped aside from in order to allow him entry. Yet, even in this case, it says something about the man's courage (and/or his utter lack of hope or power—but courage, still, in the condition of hopelessness), that despite his fearful and dreadful delusional beliefs, he entered the room and allowed himself to be locked in with the MHO. Hence, and in passing, if this and other of the author's similar experiences count as evidence, a disturbed man or woman can retain and make manifest some essential personal integrity, heroic stoicism, or an inner manifestation of 'health' that even severe mental disturbance cannot wrest from them. Sacks (quoted in Seedhouse, 2001) puts it as follows: he 'draws on a strength unfathomable to me, a [metaphysical state of] health which [was] deeper than the depth of [his] illness' (p. 50).

TENTATIVE OBSERVING

So, the MHO can begin to make tentative observations about the mental state of each new Tenaray; this, with regard to each Tenaray's posture, gait and, yes, eye contact (or lack of eye contact), or agitated eye movements. These details provide initial indicators of an individual's engagement with his/her surroundings, their psycho-emotional response to their situation. After all, the overnight incarceration and the relative seriousness of the charges, along with the advance toward day and the opening of the courts, may, even without any other factors being present, reasonably be expected to impact on a person's sense of well-being or emotional equilibrium. The strange surroundings and the stimulus that comes with knowing or unknowing 'anticipation' may produce observable levels of anxiety, agitation, annoyance, anger, or, in the case of a deeply disturbed mind, anything between and including the fight-or-flight impulse, or fearful incomprehension. Some of these observations and impressions are subtle, while others are less so.

Our Tenaray, the one charged with the theft of brie and grape sandwiches, and who joked about Manchester United with his Escort, appears to be utterly unflustered by his current surroundings and circumstances. Indeed, one could quite easily start making assumptions about how familiar this situation was for Tenaray (perhaps over more than four successive days). But let's not do that! Let's just accept that Tenaray's observed behaviour might be indicative of a certain mood or mental state, and that this impression, along with any others obtained thus far (e.g. including the seeming irrational insistence, on the part of this author's Judas Eye, that there's something 'disturbing' about this particular Tenaray), must be set aside pending the establishment of a relationship or perceptual dialogue with Tenaray.

PHENOMENOLOGY: ISSUES OF PERCEPTION AND MEANING OR 'THE EYE IN THE MIND'S SKY' (SOKOLOWSKI, 2000)

[L]ooking involves a kind of oscillation. (Baudrillard, 1988: 24)

Levin (1999), in describing what he terms, 'Descartes' Window', discusses how, with Descartes, the eye becomes a window on 'the world outside'. This conception of what the eye is and what it does confirms and appears to make concrete or factual, the ideas of interiority (i.e. as '"a visceral sense of insideness", the sense of self carried within' [Sidlauskas, 2000: 77] and exteriority, of an isolated inner self and an externality inhabited by aliens, or at least people who are forever 'unknowable' and who are, in turn, incapable of knowing one's own interiority). According to this perspective, the objective eye isolates each one of us in our skulls—creating a distance between each of us and our familiars, and preventing us from 'being-in-the-world'. This is the view from Descartes' Window, from where other people become 'moving hats and coats', automatons, solipsist toys, or aliens.

For phenomenologists, though, the eye is much more than a passive, one-way-only, 'scientific instrument' for objectively observing the outside world. Indeed, the phenomenological eye is regarded as an arbitrational instrument, a portal or corridor for the transmission and reception of data and information between alleged 'mental interiors' and external objects 'in the world'. Hence, even if one cannot disabuse oneself entirely of the either/or notions of interiority-exteriority—indeed, the author actually employs precisely this model or convention in attempting, at the same time, to question it—there is, in The Phenomenologist's Eye, the potential for the exploration of the so-called 'interiors of Others', as well as for having one's own relative interiority explored by Others. In this way, we are at once freed of our isolation (i.e. behind the curtained window of our eye) and our solipsistic sense of alienation, but at the cost, perhaps, of being capable of being 'known' by a co-existing Other. Such knowledge, whether perceived of as being a threat to the uniqueness of the individual, or as an opportunity for increasing our understanding of one another, would have been impossible for Descartes. Hence,

> [T]he right state of mind for a [phenomenologically orientated] philosopher is an active looking-both-ways, outward and inward simultaneously. (Wilson, 1976: 99)

However, Cartesian dualism, with its bipolar concepts of interiority (i.e. ethereal unreality) and exteriority (i.e. physical reality), of Mind and Body, has an enduring and deeply entrenched cognitive and social currency. In terms of perception, the Cartesian world-view has resulted in, for this writer, a dubious split between what have been termed 'primary' and 'secondary' perceptual qualities. This perceptual split involves the idea that primary qualities of perception are those that relate to matter observed, to physical objects in the external world. Primary qualities are capable of being touched and/or measured. Secondary qualities 'are where the primary ones are; they attach to the physical object' (Miller, 1973: 135), but they are of a qualitatively different, 'at a distance', order of experience. Secondary qualities, according to Miller (1973), can be perceived 'in' a person or object, but they can't be touched or objectively weighed or measured. These secondary qualities have no spatio-temporal reality (i.e. they are qualities that the observer superimposes upon, or in other ways imbues 'into', the object or person that comes under their gaze).

This distinction between primary and secondary quality perceiving is well illustrated in Sartre's (Aronson, 1980) discussion of aesthetics and, in particular, in relation to an encounter with a specific painting (i.e. Brueghel's 'The Wedding Dance'). Although Sartre doesn't couch the discussion in terms of primary and secondary qualities, his understanding of the types of perception involved is relevant. For, when stood in front of the painting, what would the primary quality observer actually *see*? According to Sartre, the answer would be: 'the glass covering it [i.e. the painting], the strokes of colour, the lines, the frame' (Sartre, cited in Aronson, 1980). Sartre goes on:

> [T]he scene appeared only when I assumed the imaginary attitude, and so created a synthetic imaginative whole that was not before me but was, strictly speaking, present only in my mind. Yet I did not seem to perform any special activity in seeing [the painting]. I did not feel more active or more spontaneous, I did not seem to be imagining rather than looking. Indeed I seemed precisely to be experiencing the object directly before me, and not something else,

something unreal. Now, I am in fact spontaneous and creative when I see a painting—but when I look away from it I realize that I must be so in order to see *anything*. Turning to the grey chair behind me, I must sort and synthesize in order for the chair to appear. Passive optical registration of what is present would give me only an incoherent jumble of unknowns. In order to *see* anything, I must also think and imagine. (Ibid: 62)

Sartre's example and explanation of 'the imaginative attitude' is adopted, here, as a good description of how inseparable primary quality perceptions (i.e. smears of paint on canvas) are from their secondary quality counterparts (i.e. the meaning-content of the painting), and of how 'the healing of the split', if, indeed, there is one, applies as much to the world of the everyday as it does in an art gallery. How strange, then, that it is precisely these secondary, 'imaginative' qualities that objective scientists/observers seek to purge from the world-laboratory of facts and truths.

Nevertheless, even if one were to insist on the existence of these primary and secondary distinctions within the act of perceiving, one would also have to accept, on the current argument, that there is a sense in which the one is utterly dependent upon the other. That is, 'Perception presents me with a spectacle as varied and as clearly articulated as possible' (Merleau-Ponty, 2005: 292), but the quality or nature of that perception is mediated by our past experiences and current attitudes. For example, if I were a creature capable only of perceiving primary qualities (i.e. the painted surface/person as object, but not its/his essential 'meaning-content'), what would I actually *see* in Tenaray's actions and movements toward me? A moving organism, perhaps, or an 'It', a moving substance or 'a something', or matter undifferentiated from the other matter that fills vision (except, perhaps, by something called Movement)? Bereft of secondary qualities, my perception might be objective, and accurate up to a point, but it would be barren of significant human content and meaning (e.g. I, and not just the I-as-MHO, would be incapable of recognising, in Tenaray's act of walking towards me, the plethora of co-existent meanings that attend the activity, and so, arguably, would be unable to distinguish between threatening and non-threatening non-verbal behaviour, shame or haughtiness). Indeed, one could argue that such an objective primary quality perception is, if it could be extruded out of meaning at all, a one-eyed absurdity. Certainly, such a singular focus would be a distinct liability in a magistrate's cells. Put bluntly, behaviour must be 'read' or interpreted—it has to have a meaningful context (i.e. either situationally and/or compared to something else) in order to be understood. Hence, a primary quality perception might be objectively true (whatever 'Truth' is), but any claim as to the authenticity of such observations, and to any substantial truth (i.e. by social human beings) about what, exactly, is happening in any human behaviour, interaction, or encounter, is mandated upon the so-called secondary quality perception-meanings being 'enmeshed' in, or coterminous with, primary quality perception.

Hence, the perceiving eye, the eye as interior-exterior arbitrator, has to oscillate between 'eye as objective observing-measuring instrument'—though an instrument with no markings or scales—and 'eye influenced by secondary qualities'. These secondary qualities may, in turn, have their root in, and be influenced by, the workings of The Judas Eye.

For, if inferences, as secondary quality functions, cannot be made, then the concept of 'assessment', as an 'evaluation of the merits of a person or object' (Irvine, 1971), becomes utterly redundant (i.e. since the 'evaluation of merits' is a decidedly secondary quality activity).

Hence, an assessment of an individual's merits, with regard to their mental health, necessitates a process whereby the observed person (i.e. Tenaray) is meaningfully perceived by the MHO. So, and without engaging in a distracting overview of the philosophy of mind with regard to Others (Glendinning, 1999), and of consciousness in particular (Chalmers, 1996), a brief outline of how this eye-to-eye encounter could be experienced may aid the reader's understanding. To this end, Valéry's model of 'the gaze' (cited in Freedman, 1991) makes an interesting and, for this writer, accurate starting point. For Valéry, then, 'once gazes interlock, there are no longer *quite* two persons and it's hard for either to remain *alone*'. In short, the encounter consists of a chiasmatic intersecting of two 'lifelines', two viewpoints, creating a unit of 'we' (what Sartre [2003], calls '*Mitsein*' or 'Being-With'). You take my appearance, my image (or at least the I-as-MHO's image), and I take yours (or at least the image of 'Tenaray-the-incarcerated' that Tenaray elects to bring or project into this particular encounter). This 'taking of one another's image', within 'the gaze', is explored in greater depth under the heading of 'the pre-verbal relational dyad' (below). However, I would ask the reader to begin to consider how each of us might attempt to evaluate the merits of The Other by reference to, say, primary and secondary qualities, and in terms of the extent to which we are allowed, or in other ways gain access to, The Other's perceived interiority.

In the meantime, though, the conversation between Tenaray and his Escort has reached a seemingly natural end. Tenaray begins to turn his attention to this new space, the cell space area. He begins to turn and lift his head in the MHO's direction. He appears to be aware of the fact that he is 'being observed', but he has not yet set eyes on the MHO.

A PHILOSOPHICAL-PHENOMENOLOGICAL PLACE FOR THE I AND I-AS-MHO TO STAND

Phenomenology is the study of the way things appear to us in experience or consciousness (Sokolowski, 2000). Phenomenology is less to do with the study of objects or facts, and more to do with the study of events as they appear in our experience. Phenomenology seeks to describe experience without being obstructed (or mediated) by preconceptions, theoretical ideas, and personal prejudices (Moran, 2000). Furthermore, 'Phenomenology has to interrogate the supposedly objective views of the sciences, what has been termed the "God's eye" perspective, or the "view from nowhere"' (Moran, 2000: 12). The act of looking, of *seeing*, is, for the phenomenologist, the critical-analytical process whereby he or she discovers the mutual relatedness of subjectivity and objectivity (e.g. of the alleged primary and secondary qualities of perception), of interiority and exteriority, of his or her sense of personal identity within the dynamic context of relationships with Others, and with the world of ideas and objects:

> Everything has appearance and essence, shell and kernel, mask and truth. What does it say against the inward determination of things that we finger the shell without reading the kernel, that we live with appearance instead of perceiving the essence, that the mask of things so blinds us that we cannot find the truth? (Marc, cited in Chipp, 1968: 449–50)

Hence, given the author's confessed bias towards a seeking-after both 'the shell' of appearance and 'the kernel' of truth in the act of perceiving, it will come as no surprise to the reader that the author looks to phenomenology when seeking to describe and discuss his encounters with any Tenaray.

Phenomenology posits two basic forms of perception. The first, the 'natural attitude' is the default position for living (i.e. we see what we need to see in order to get on with the tasks of daily living—though not automatons or zombies, we are, nevertheless, preoccupied with actions, tasks, and commitments). One example of how phenomenologists conceive the natural attitude mode of experiencing is provided by Depraz (in Fulford, et al, 2003), where she states that it is:

> situated on the plane of ... everydayness and familiarity. [This] implies that, on the one hand, [such experiences] often pass unnoticed because they go without saying for us. On the other hand, these experiences derive meaning from repetition and ritualization and, therefore, from their sedimentation into the individual history of each person. (p. 190)

The second form of perception is the 'phenomenological attitude'. The phenomenological attitude, put bluntly, is when, in our reflected consciousness, we 'think about thinking', when we (as far as we are capable) suspend our prejudices, when we consciously attend to, and open ourselves to being 'innocently/tranquilly receptive' of the objects of our perception. For phenomenologists, this shift in conscious thought or attending, this break with the default position of our natural flow of lived experiences, constitutes an actual 'rupturing' (Depraz, 2003) of the natural attitude. The phenomenological attitude can be imposed upon us (e.g. by an exceptional, violent, or unexpected and rather singular event), or we can elect to attend to an object, person, or event from within the phenomenological attitude. Even so, such an 'innocent receptivity' is a state-of-being not so easily acquired. For, with the search for objective or scientific 'truths' appearing to have achieved the status of 'a religion', one can begin to understand how:

the very activity of sense perception has nowhere to go in a world in which science deals with ideal qualities, and comes to have little enough exchange value in a money market dominated by considerations of calculation, measurement, profit and the like. (Jameson, cited in Jay, 1994: 153)

That said, this entire chapter is the product of the author's reflections on his own experience of employing the phenomenological attitude, more or less successfully, in the setting and circumstances described.

THE SECRETING-AWAY OF 'IDOLS' (IN SECONDARY QUALITY PERCEIVING)

So, in order to even attempt to move towards a state of innocent receptivity, I (i.e. not merely the I-as-MHO) must exorcise a number of what Bacon (cited in Seedhouse, 2001) termed 'Idols':

> The idols have seen lots of poverty,
> Snakes and gold and lice,
> But not the truth.
> (Wallace Stevens, cited in Levin, 1999: 420)

These Idols are hidden in the so-called secondary quality perceptions. They are part of what one 'imbues into' one's perception of a person or object, but they also have the potential to skew one's perception. These Idols are defined by Seedhouse (2001) as:

> the *Idols of the Tribe* (i.e. our 'tendency to suppose that our senses give full and accurate knowledge of reality'); of the *Cave* (i.e. 'our personal biases ... [based on] our unique experiences [and beliefs]'); of the *Theatre* (i.e. ideas that 'have immigrated into men's minds from the various dogmas of philosophies'. (Bacon, cited in Seedhouse, 2001: pp. 25–6)

> and of the *Market Place* (i.e. 'the errors which result from the communication and association of men with each other.'). (Solzhenitsyn, cited in Seedhouse, 2001: 26)

These authors argue that these Idols, our individual Idols, enslave our Thought, funnelling it into a bland acceptance of 'the shells of appearance', of materialism, functionalism, and positivism, and, consequently, of a pseudo-shallow form of thinking that, often, isn't even our own examined Thought. Also, although not addressed at all in this paper, the problem of unexamined Idols could also be extended to include the 'meaning-made-manifest' of the (Freudian?) Unconscious, as well as Gladwell's (2005) and Kihlstrom's (1996) concept of, respectively, the Adaptive Unconscious and The Judas Eye.

So, having elected to adopt or 'enter' the phenomenological attitude, I now have the task of constructing an I-as-MHO with a mental state-of-being that is, as far as possible, stripped of such layers and 'infestations' of idolatry as my self-knowledge or 'personal knowing' (Carper, 1978, and cited in White, 1997), and mental discipline can realistically achieve and maintain. This mental state-of-being also has to have, as its visual correlate (remembering my commitment to the physical manifesting of a 'tranquil receptivity'), a genuine 'physico-psycho-emotional openness' with regard to the imminent encounter with Tenaray: 'Each moment demands of me the labour of my own will' (Johnson, 1971: 2).

The mental act of interrogating one's own secondary quality perceptions, with a view to identifying and eradicating (or at least recognising) idolatrous features is not, as the author has already attempted to demonstrate, something that can be easily or even wholly achieved—since, for this writer, to perceive is, concurrently-simultaneously, to *see* meaning in what is perceived (or, if meaning does *follow* perception—as Kihlstrom (1996) and the primary-secondary perceptual model suggest—then the 'space' and/or oscillations between the two are not always immediately before our consciousness). However, the 'perception-meaning' and 'primary-secondary quality' arguments or dialectics are not the only barriers to an ideal mode of perceiving or an innocent receptivity. There is, too, the deeply entrenched—at least in the West—psychology of the unconscious self/selves (to be sharply distinguished from the Adaptive Unconscious/The Judas Eye), an endless succession of, seemingly, secreted-away 'darker selves', wherein, as the last of a succession of smaller and smaller Russian dolls, there resides an unknowable but utterly loathsome creature; a creature, so the mythology goes, 'teeming in the silence of repression' (Baudrillard, 1988: 24). This is a Gollum-like creature that last saw the light of the sun in some primordial swamp.

So, the MHO has to 'set' himself to keeping one eye on Tenaray's presenting unification of primary and secondary qualities (i.e. his personage or 'thing-ness' as he traverses the physical space between himself and the doorframe/MHO). This setting of one aspect of Self, as a condition of the I-as-MHO's role, brings with it a further 'perception-meanings' complication. For, 'whenever the process of simple perception and bare apprehension passes over into that of inspection and scrutiny', a checklist of 'self-instructions appear' (Vernon, 1937: 45). If one accepts that the MHO's state-of-being includes the role of an inspector and scrutiniser, then one could reasonably expect that such a state-of-being would be at odds with one's quest for an innocent receptivity and, possibly, damaging of the phenomenological attitude itself. However, this aspect of the MHO's role is here regarded as an 'oscillation destination' (i.e. one of a number of more 'primary quality-orientated' shifts in the mode of perceiving, but with each mode including its own instructions/checklist), as part of a 'multi-layered concurrent simultaneity'—that actually enriches the experience of experiencing.

Also, and at one and the same time as the MHO observes with a 'risk' checklist in mind, the second eye is immersed in and guided by a relative state of 'innocent receptivity' (i.e. supposedly bereft of Idols, [relatively] unencumbered by the positive or negative impressions of The Judas Eye, and 'free' of our individual Gollum-esque insecurities) within the phenomenological attitude. All this, while retaining a certain (professional and personal) 'curiosity' as to what exchanges may or may not occur in One Another's gaze into the Cartesian 'window-eyes' of The Other.

Such oscillations between modes of perceiving, or such a deluge of 'concurrent simultaneity' of Perceptions (Scheler, 1954), demand considerable self-knowledge, cognitive discipline, and an understanding of how, for oneself at least, and in this situation, 'meaning' is co-existent or coterminous with 'perception'.

In any event, Tenaray and his Escort are eight paces away. Tenaray has now fixed his gaze on the MHO's shoes, trousers, shirt. I note that, as Tenaray's face is coming up to meet mine, he has five or six fresh stitches in an ugly cut under his left eye. This cut runs vertically down his cheek, with the last stitch tugging at the corner of his mouth, forcing his features into what looked like a sneer. The two sides of the wound were roughly drawn together. The taut black threads and knots appear to evidence a sewing-hand guided by haste and utility rather than any sound professional or cosmetic aesthetic (i.e. either the suture nurse was blindfolded at the time of the sewing, or, perhaps, Tenaray was 'non-compliant' with the treatment being offered, or both). The flesh around the eye is swollen and his cheek looks misshapen, asymmetrical within the geometries of his face. Nevertheless, I instantly recognise him as someone I assessed many years ago. The sense of unease that Memory and The Judas Eye had earlier produced now conference a sudden chill, a chill that quickly gives way to the forming of a word-concept. The word-concept is 'evil-ness'. Innocent receptivity is at once impaled on the word-concept. The carefully and delicately constructed cradle of the phenomenological attitude is tipped into oblivion. Memory 'fills in the blanks' (with half-forgotten facts). Tenaray-is-evil, evil-is-Tenaray! This new knowledge calls for an urgent reframing. The word-concept needs, somehow, to be suspended, removed from thinking. Yet how, I ask myself, does one instruct oneself to forget, to order oneself not to think, for example, of the colour blue? For the simple instruction itself ensures that, even if blue were not 'before my mind's eye' to begin with, it is now.

Tenaray, or Omo-Tenaray as I will call this 'new' Tenaray, has changed his name and put on weight, but he is undoubtedly the same man who, all those years ago, was eventually sent to prison for stalking and raping the woman who had been his History teacher. The same Omo-Tenaray, who, as part of a plea bargaining, had also admitted to a series of similar offences.

Omo-Tenaray and I are an instant away from making eye contact with one another, and the I-as-MHO suddenly has the task of absorbing and then suspending this new information. With the I-as-MHO almost overcome by all kinds of unhelpful moral and value judgements, the 'I', at least, recognises that all kinds of Idols are afoot and in clear view, and that an urgent 'clearing-out' needs to be undertaken:

> Perception involves the active and passive processes of the interpretation of information ... Prejudice involves judgements and opinions formed without due examination of relevant information (i.e. making assumptions). (Towl & Crighton, 1996: 63)

Clearly, the situation in the cells is less than ideal. Indeed, and as has just been demonstrated, there is the potential for all manner of bias and prejudice, stereotyping and labelling, misunderstanding and misperceptions, on either or both sides. In short, the environment would appear to contain all the necessary ingredients in which Idols could prosper. However, it is precisely because the environment is so 'Idol-friendly' that issues surrounding how one perceives, including one's own awareness of one's perceptual prejudices, and, crucially, how one could be or is likely to be perceived by The Other, come before one's own mind for examination, censure, or re-adoption.

Crudely, then, it would seem that both I and the I-as-MHO have to attain and maintain, or at least oscillate between, at least two seemingly contradictory perceptual states-of-being (i.e. in this instance, the 'informed' and somewhat jaundiced Judas Eye, with the checklist observer at his shoulder, and the relatively innocent phenomenological eye). This, while concurrently-simultaneously presenting a relaxed and open posture, mentally guarding against potential sabotage from 'within' (i.e. one's conscious prejudices or Idols; the play or downright mischief of some vague but strangely 'sensed' Unconscious Self [or Selves]; and whatever well-meaningness one can extrude from The Judas Eye), and inspecting or scrutinising what lies 'without' with an at once open but analytical gaze.

Hence, the MHO has much to consider in the 'just standing stood there' moments that precede the establishing of eye contact with Omo-Tenaray. Omo-Tenaray's head is now almost fully lifted—his gaze travels up my neck and chin—but the MHO is struggling. Struggling with memories of the stalking-and-rape case. Struggling to decide what to do if Omo-Tenaray recognises his old assessor, or what to do or say if he doesn't.

Calm, calm, calm! One mustn't judge or pre-judge. Where's that tranquil receptivity so recently acquired, that fragile structure, so strenuously constructed? Is it within reach? Is it to be found at all? … There, there it is! I can see it! Now, if I can but reach out and grasp it.

So, Omo-Tenaray's eyes meet with mine. This is a defining moment, a moment, if you like, of praxis (i.e. where knowledge and meaning are constructed out of experience). The mutual gaze, a pre-verbal relational dyad, is thus engaged. Forget everything else! For this is the moment towards which all else has, for the MHO, been sculpted and directed. Primary and secondary qualities function concurrently-simultaneously; The Judas Eye does its work—though with a 'values-monitor' rigorously analysing and interpreting both what has been meaningfully perceived and what has been 'pressed' into (visual) metaphor; the interlocked gaze creates a system consisting of two people relating to one another in congruent participation, in such a way that, and again, 'there are no longer *quite* two persons and it's hard for either to remain *alone*' (Merleau-Ponty citing Valéry, in Freedman, 1991: 65).

Anyway, and for the moment, let us assume that the MHO is 'in' the phenomenological attitude, or taking the 'view from nowhere' (Moran, 2000), together with what the author has described as 'a tranquil receptivity', and that the mutual relatedness of subjectivity and objectivity, of interiority and exteriority, allow of a two-way exploration of The Other that doesn't stop at the cornea or the iris. In short, the gaze involves mutual thin-slicing on all sorts of levels, so that The One 'creates' The Other for himself in his own 'mind's eye'.

So, a two-way visual communication corridor is opened up. I see the flicker of recognition in Omo-Tenaray's eyes and face. His face betrays the smile that indicates that his recollection of me is a positive one. The 'I' sighs with relief. At least the 'minefield' of reintroductions and reminding doesn't appear to be a problem. There is, too, his smile—a positive platform from which we can both negotiate and build or re-build a relationship.

Omo-Tenaray appears to have processed his previous memories of the I-as-MHO and he wears those recollections on his face, in a seemingly genuine but at the same time twisted (i.e. due to the pull of the stitches), almost sneering smile. In accepting these facial movements as a genuine smile, rather than as a sneer, the author brings past experience and a little idolatry—if 'optimism' is a bias—to the negotiating table. So, Omo-Tenaray's smile seems to confirm that the MHO's manifesting of a non-judgemental tranquil receptivity has 'worked'. At least, that is, in the early nano-seconds of the dyad. Hence, in bringing genuine aspects of Self to the role of the I-as-MHO, the actor's skills would seem to have been vindicated. That said, the potential 'trap', for the 'I' and the I-as-MHO, is not so much in the area of 'observing' what can be seen and/or measured (e.g. speed of walking), but in misperceiving or misinterpreting the so-called secondary quality content (e.g. Omo-Tenaray's smile or misperceiving or misinterpreting the meaning and content that is conveyed in 'the gaze').

The MHO's non-threatening gaze is intended as 'an offer' of human contact and, in this case, familiarity, toward Omo-Tenaray. Omo-Tenaray, for his part is now gazing intently at the MHO. While the MHO's direct gaze is a targeted transmission to Omo-Tenaray, there is also the matter of the jaundiced eye—trying (unsuccessfully) to remain primary quality focused and gathering together physical observations or data about Omo-Tenaray's physical co-ordination and functioning within the situational context.

With the pre-verbal relational dyad or two-way visual corridor functioning, the encounter, proper, commences.

EYE CONTACT, BRACKETING, PRESENCING, AND THE ELASTICITY OF TIME

[The] immediacy [of the experience] knows neither exact space nor objective time and causality. (Moran, citing Husserl's *Experience and Judgement* [1938], 2000: 12)

'For Heidegger the present, the now, is not a measurable unit of time, but the result of a presence, of the existent actively presenting itself' (Berger, 1980: 86). This 'nowness' or '*presencing*' (Heidegger, cited in Berger, 1980, and Heidegger, 2003) has, in the context of the pre-verbal relational dyad or visual two-way corridor (i.e. direct eye-to-eye contact and mutual relating), a curious impact on time itself. For time, as marked by the clock, as measurable units or periods in linear and constant flow, can slow and stall. For, with eye-to-eye contact having once been engaged, the encounter, the pre-verbal relational dyad could acquire a seeming 'tempo, ... duration', and 'sequen(tial)' (Lauer, in Thiselton, 1999) life of its own. Arguably, a relational dyad could be perceived to consist of a 'creaturely' (Thistelton, 1999) or 'human-interactive' dialogue that stands outside of natural clock-time. This capsule of phenomenological experiencing, though bracketed between clock-time (e.g. clock-time being suspended when eye contact is made, and beginning again once eye contact is broken), has the potential to contain a number of timeframes and inner journeys, for both parties, that are removed from the clock's measured ticking-off of each step Omo-Tenaray takes. Within this dyad, this embryonic relating, the concept of clock-time, can appear to become suspended or, even, redundant.

The nature and quality of this initial eye-to-eye transaction may well determine whether or not Omo-Tenaray will consent to any form of mental health assessment. Hence, it is essential that the MHO communicate openness (on several levels), amenability, self-assuredness, and acceptance, of The Other, in those instants of silent communion. The MHO has to provide the visual credentials of genuineness, professional authority, and unconditional positive regard that will secure a basic level of trust and so prepare the way for constructive verbal communication. This is very often much easier said than done. For instance, the MHO may have obtained full details of some of Omo-Tenaray's full offending history, as well as, often, graphic written accounts (e.g. from the injured party or from a series of witnesses) of the current alleged offence. This prior knowledge, though essential to establishing any potential risk factors in advance of the assessment, can expose the MHO to prejudicial influences which, unless the 'I' behind the I-as-MHO has a highly developed awareness of self, could form negative preconceptions and misconceptions (i.e. allowing Idols to dominate) even before meeting this or that Omo-Tenaray.

In terms of an initial assessment of risk, this silent eye-to-eye transaction is of vital importance. For, if eye contact is not made (e.g. the potential assessee stares fixedly at the floor or, in the case of one individual who appeared to be experiencing visual hallucinations, was staring from side to side, up and down, behind him, and over the my shoulder, as if someone were stood behind me), then one faces the prospect of being locked in a room with someone with whom no 'eye-to-eye relationship' has been established and in relation to whom one might have serious misgivings about trying to assess with any degree of safety. The safety issue is not merely with regard to one's own personal safety, as there is also the need to make a rapid judgement about the levels of vulnerability or distress of the prospective assessee (e.g. an already frightened individual, on the edge of the flight or fight impulse, may, on being locked in a room with a complete stranger, be 'driven' to act one way or another).

'IN A DARK TIME, THE EYE BEGINS TO SEE'
(ROETHKE, 1966)

> Such is the gaze, whose force resides precisely in it not being an exchange, but a double moment, a double mark, immediate, undecipherable. (Baudrillard, 1988: 61)

There have been a very few occasions when, with eye contact engaged, the prospective Tenaray has, either by intent or through some disability or disorder, been unwilling or unable to enter into a qualitative eye-to-eye transaction that involved the transmission and receipt of layers of information and emotional meaning. There have also been instances where the prospective Tenaray has, while looking the author straight in the eye, intended that no transaction, interaction, or exchange would take place. This was often communicated by an intense or hostile glance or stare (e.g. a one-way transmission that trumpets a 'no entry!' or a 'don't even try it!'). Nietzsche wrote that:

> He who fights with monsters should look to it that he himself does not become a monster ... And when you gaze long into an abyss, the abyss also gazes into you. (Nietzsche, 1990: 102)

More chilling, though, is the eye-to-eye 'engagement' wherein no intense or hostile barriers are erected, no discernible psycho-emotional guards are in place, and the I-as-MHO journeys into the desolate wilderness of a crushed spirit, or the savagely gnarled ennui of an under-controlled or, even more unnerving, an over-controlled psychopathic mind. In these last cases, where a 'Shark's Eye' or a 'Dead Eye', or a 'Medusan Eye' (i.e. the seeming intent [or wish] is to turn one to stone), is presented, there is often no dialogue (unless 'no dialogue' counts as a dialogue), no negotiation, only an existential journey which, and at the risk of being overly dramatic, sees the traveller peering into Nietzsche's abyss. Indeed, some of these revealed landscapes are very dark places, and the MHO needs to be acutely aware of what could occur if his/her curiosity were to get the better of them and they decided 'to go exploring'. For, by undertaking such an expedition, the MHO necessarily suspends his/her peripheral vision, their (supposedly primary quality) looking and observing in the 'outside world', and unconsciously exposes their own gaze—their 'unguarded gaze'—to the view of someone whose skills of character recognition and analysis may very well be superior to those of the I-as-MHO's, or even the I's, now, 'unguarded inner feeling-landscapes'.

How, though, do I presume to begin to make inferences based on variable types of eye contact and the time it takes to traverse a distance of ten paces? Well, and assuming Omo-Tenaray has made and engaged in some level of eye contact, there are the transactions that took place within the pre-verbal relational dyad (i.e. the silent but mutual giving and receiving of non-verbal communications between Omo-Tenaray and myself).

EXPERIENCING WITHIN THE PRE-VERBAL RELATIONAL DYAD

> It is never when eyes are looking at you that you can find them beautiful or ugly, that you can remark on their colour ... The Other's look hides his eyes: he seems to go *in front of* them. (Sartre, cited in Jay, 1994: 288)

For the author, pre-verbal relational dyads tend to involve 'oscillations', a conscious switching of perceptions between objective peripheral vision and subjective perceiving (e.g. involving my own metaphorical and analogous imaginings). Such 'feeling-landscapes' are then interpreted, not sequentially, but en masse or in toto. Though this means of perceiving conveys no literal visual images or imaginings, the resulting perception is, nevertheless, *like* a landscape. When the author looks into the eyes of an Other, any Other, my inner perceptions of what that Other eye conveys, either directly, or via access gained or denied within our eye negotiations, tends to reveal itself to me, in my experiencing, as a feeling-landscape. The experience of each of the protagonists (inner) eye, vying with the other (i.e. allowing access here, closing portals here, and gatekeeping or building an obstruction there), don't decrease the dynamism of the relational dyad, they spice it up. The experience is 'like' something—it is like.

INTERPRETATION

As far as Omo-Tenaray is concerned, my impression of his feeling-landscape(s) was one of harsh lines and barren expanses, scorched earth and icy crevasses, with many a gateway portcullis'd-up and designated 'entry forbidden'. A human being, one felt, wouldn't survive long in such a landscape. Ardrey (1967) provides an excellent addendum to this author's clichéd feeling-landscapes when, in relation to someone else, he describes:

> ... a restiveness in [the] man. It [was] unease unaware, demand undeclared, the hunger of a man at midnight who opens the refrigerator door, finds nothing that he really wants, and closing the door, goes back to bed. There is a darkening, inward, indefinite mood that retains an outward poise, like that of a box of nitroglycerine at rest. (p. 321)

In the meantime, of course, Omo-Tenaray had been surveying my inner eye, my inner portals, and forming his own impressions of the I-as-MHO.

An oscillated return to 'this reality' reveals that Omo-Tenaray's outward gaze has acquired a flinty, abrasive quality—the nitroglycerine, it seems, had been jostled from its rest.

The subjective 'truth' would appear to be that this Omo-Tenaray is no 'open book'. Certainly, he is very discriminating in what he will or won't disclose with regard to his feeling-landscapes. In any event, Omo-Tenaray has 'signalled' that the pre-verbal relational dyad is coming to an end and the I-as-MHO must set aside interpretation and reinstate the phenomenological attitude.

ENDINGS

On the tenth step: I introduce myself and observe for non-verbal cues (e.g. a nod, an 'eye-lid acknowledgement') that what I have just said has been 'received' and understood. I invite 'the subject' into the room (i.e. usually with an open gesture of the arm as well as verbally), and, if he chooses to enter, I follow.

REFERENCES

Ardrey, R (1967) *The Territorial Imperative: A personal inquiry into the animal origins of property and nations.* London: Collins.
Aronson, R (1980) *Jean-Paul Sartre: Philosophy in the world.* London: NLB and Verso Editions.
Baudrillard, J (1988) *The Ecstasy of Communication* S Lotringer (Ed) (B Schutze & C Schutze, Trans). New York: Semiotext(e).
Benner, P (1984) *From Novice to Expert: Excellence and power in clinical nursing practice.* Menlo Park, CA: Addison-Wesley.
Berger, J (1980) *About Looking.* London: Writers and Readers Publishing Cooperative.
Burnard, P (2003) Ordinary chat and therapeutic conversations: Phatic communication and mental health nursing. *Journal of Psychiatric and Mental Health Nursing, 10* (6), 678–82.
Carper, B (1978) Fundamental patterns of knowing. *Advanced Nursing Science, 1* (1), 13–23.
Chalmers, DJ (1996) *The Conscious Mind: In search of a fundamental theory.* Oxford: Oxford University Press.
Chipp, HB (1968) *Theories of Modern Art.* Berkeley, CA/Los Angeles, CA: University of California.
Department of Health and Social Security (1983) *Mental Health Act 1983: Memorandum on Parts I to VI, VIII and X.* London: HMSO.
Depraz, N (2003) Putting the *épochè* into practice: Schizophrenic experience as illustrating the phenomenological exploration of consciousness. In B Fulford, K Morris, JZ Sadler & G Stanghellini (Eds) *Nature and Narrative: An introduction to the new philosophy of psychiatry* (pp 187–98). Oxford: Oxford University Press.
Freedman, B (1991) *Staging the Gaze: Postmodernism, psychoanalysis, and Shakespearean comedy.* London: Cornell University Press.
Gladwell, M (2005) *Blink: The power of thinking without thinking.* London: Allen Lane/Penguin Books.
Glendinning, S (1999) *On Being with Others: Heidegger – Derrida – Wittgenstein.* London: Routledge.
Heidegger, M (2003) *Being and Time* (J Macquarrie & E Robinson, Trans). Oxford: Blackwell.
Henle, M (1961) *Documents of Gestalt Psychology.* Berkeley, CA: University of California.
Irvine, AH (Ed) (1971) *Collins New English Dictionary.* London: Collins.
Jay, M (1994) *Downcast Eyes: The denigration of vision in twentieth century French thought.* London: University of California Press.
Johnson, RE (1971) *Existential Man: The challenge of psychotherapy.* New York: Pergamon.
Kihlstrom, JF (1996) Perception without awareness of what is perceived, learning without awareness of what is learned. In M Velmans (Ed) *The Science of Consciousness: Psychological, neuropsychological and clinical reviews* (pp 21–46). London: Routledge.

Levin, DM (1999) *The Philosopher's Gaze: Modernity in the shadows of enlightenment.* London: University of California Press.
Malinowski, B (1922) *Argonauts of the Western Pacific: An account of native enterprise and adventure in the archipelago of Melanesian New Guinea.* London: Routledge.
Merleau-Ponty, M (2005) *Phenomenology of Perception* (C Smith, Trans). Abingdon: Routledge.
Miller, DL (1973) *George Herbert Mead: Self, language and the world.* Chicago: University of Chicago Press.
Moran, D (2000) *Introduction to Phenomenology.* London: Routledge.
Nagel, T (1995) *Other Minds: Critical essays 1969–1994.* Oxford: Oxford University Press.
Nietzsche, F (1990) *Beyond Good and Evil: Prelude to a philosophy of the future.* (RJ Hollingdale, Trans). London: Penguin.
Roethke, T (1966*) The Collected Poems of Theodore Roethke: In a dark time.* London: Faber & Faber.
Sartre, JP (2003) *Being and Nothingness* (HE Barnes, Trans). Abingdon: Routledge Classics.
Scheler, M (1954) *The Nature of Sympathy* (P Heath, Trans). London: Routledge.
Seedhouse, D (2001) *Health: The foundations for achievement* (2nd edn). Chichester: Wiley.
Sidlauskas, S (2000) *Body, Place and Self in Nineteenth-Century Painting.* Cambridge: Cambridge University Press.
Silverman, J, Kurtz, S & Draper, J (1998) *Skills for Communicating with Patients.* Abingdon: Radcliffe Medical Press.
Sokolowski, R (2000) *Introduction to Phenomenology.* Cambridge: Cambridge University Press.
Thiselton, AC (1999) Communicative action and promise in hermeneutics. In R Lundin, C Walhout & AC Thiselton *The Promise of Hermeneutics* (pp 133–239). Cambridge: Paternoster Press.
Towl, GJ & Crighton, DA (1996) *The Handbook of Psychology for Forensic Practitioners.* London: Routledge.
Vernon, MD (1937) *Visual Perception.* Cambridge: Cambridge University Press.
White, S (1997) Empathy: a literature review and concept analysis. *Journal of Clinical Nursing, 6,* 253–7.
Whittington, R & Patterson, P (1996) Verbal and non-verbal behaviour immediately prior to aggression by mentally disordered people: Enhancing the assessment of risk. *Journal of Psychiatric and Mental Health Nursing, 3,* 47–54.
Wiedenbach, E (1985) *Clinical Nursing: A helping out.* New York: Springer-Verlag.
Wilson, C (1976) *The Strength to Dream: Literature and the imagination.* London: Sphere Books.

CHAPTER 12

OPENING UP SPACE FOR DISSENSION
A QUESTIONING PSYCHOLOGY

BOB DIAMOND

As a clinical psychologist working in predominantly psychiatric mental health services, it is my view that critical theory is often dismissed as being unhelpful or simply gratuitous and irrelevant. In this chapter I will consider that sometimes, in fact more often than not, we can only be helpful when we are also critical. Throughout the chapter I will refer to both psychiatry and clinical psychology in the National Health Service (NHS). The first half of the chapter takes a critical look at practice by considering concepts of power, values and interests, and the second half considers what I suggest are more transparent and constructive frameworks for practice. I will also draw on some ideas from my own practice that stem from these influences.

WHY BE CRITICAL?

I suppose simply because so much of what we do in Psychiatric and Clinical Psychological Adult Mental Health Services doesn't seem to work. I suggest that psychiatry can be very spurious and speculative; psychotherapy, fanciful imaginative stuff and as for evidence for both, well if it were made of ice I certainly wouldn't be walking on it! These are critical views and arguably sit awkwardly with current populist approaches, however, their lack of fashionable acceptance make them no less compelling. Critical, or questioning perspectives encourage us to consider whose agenda and interests are being served within the services and who has access and influence over the wielding of power.

EVIDENCE AND PRACTICE

Double (2006) argues that although biomedical psychiatry may wish itself to be a simple, straightforward, scientific discipline, in fact the ideological nature of psychiatry and its relationship to issues of power are unavoidable. He maintains that critical thinking leads to an openness of thinking and being reflective about one's own assumptions, tolerates uncertainty and ambiguity and helps to take account of different perspectives. Psychiatry must recognise the primacy of social, cultural, economic and political contexts. Moncrieff (2006), referring to the debatable effects of psychotropic medication, considers the deficiencies in the evidence have gone largely uncommented on due to the fact that three powerful institutions (the pharmaceutical industry, the profession of psychiatry and the government) have had an interest in promoting psychiatric drug treatments and the medical and biological paradigms that usually justify and inform their use. Lynch (2006) referring to psychiatrists and GPs and the lack of evidence to equate biochemical conditions with so-called mental illness, says that there is very little evidence to back up the insistent claims that mental health problems are caused by brain abnormalities. He goes on to suggest that to acknowledge the flimsy foundations of such evidence would mean a great loss of face, respectability and status. Timimi (2006: 197) uses the term 'speculative biobabble' in summing up the clinical evidence for Attention Deficit Hyperactivity Disorder, but still this has not prevented the medicalisation of children's behaviour and the huge increase in the prescription rates of Ritalin, the preferred treatment. In the UK, prescriptions for stimulants for children have increased from about 6,000 in 1994 to about 345,000 in 2003.

Referring to psychotherapy, Epstein (2006) reviews the outcome evidence across psychotherapies and concludes that psychotherapy remains consistently ineffective. However, it persists because it reaffirms basic American values of self-sufficiency and individualism. He argues that psychotherapy should not be considered as a scientifically credible clinical discipline. Epstein describes psychotherapy as a pseudoscience and a cultural institution:

> Since all of the psychotherapeutic theories usually defy direct tests of their accuracy except through the therapies they inspire, the universal failure of clinical experiments to provide scientifically credible evidence of effective outcomes suggests that psychotherapy's major contribution is metaphoric. (p. 193)

Central to the illusion is the reliance upon belief and the power of self-invention to the extent that the illusion becomes reality in many therapies. Epstein concludes that psychotherapy has become a civil religion in North American society. Moloney (2006) notes the fact that practising psychotherapists tend to either ignore or downplay the emerging view of the limited effect of most psychotherapies and where there is an effect this is as likely to be linked to the non-specific factors in therapy. Similarly, Smail (2005) has likened psychology, on occasions, to the greatest intellectual confidence trick of the twentieth century, and a professional pursuit whose sheer economic importance should not to be underestimated.

When considering the evidence supporting the services and in particular the National Institute for Clinical Excellence (NICE), Charlton (2000) draws parallels with NHS management and the illusion of a policy sausage machine. He adds that no thinking would be necessary and all developments would be pre-determined by objective information and statistics. Charlton qualifies:

[O]f course it is all an illusion. The sausage machine is designed by politicians and operated by managers. Data input is selective, analysis is selective, and implementation is selective. The numerous political pressures and managerial judgements are shielded from critique by an elaborate façade of pseudo-evidence and quasi-mathematical impartiality. The official propaganda for NICE denies the massive role of arbitrary opinion and interest involved in deciding what *ought* to be done, and concentrates all its efforts on making people do it. (p. 25)

Taking just one example, Charlton clarifies the ethic of honesty that should permeate scientific practice; he accuses NICE of a fundamental evasiveness by conflating effectiveness with cost-effectiveness in its mission statement. In doing so, Charlton says, NICE perpetrates a basic dishonesty of implying that these quite distinct variables can be routinely satisfied by a single recommendation.

To some extent it can be argued that psychiatry and clinical psychology create their own knowledge in the interests of dominance and power; afford limited respect for individual's own views and experiences; offer explanations of illness or distress that are rooted in faults within the individual; and control the agenda for what will and will not be discussed. There are many accounts describing how such services contribute towards people's isolation and alienation, thus marginalising them further from society (Read & Reynolds, 1996; Johnstone, 2000; Wallcraft & Michaelson, 2001; Rogers & Pilgrim, 2003).

It would seem then that the substance and evidence in support of the services is much more flimsy that we may hitherto have acknowledged. I have written elsewhere (Diamond, 2004) that clinical psychology is too concerned with its own professional self-aggrandisement and have cautioned for psychology to embrace modesty and humility. Dineen (1999) considers that the psychology industry has allowed itself to be a willing, co-operative agent of social policy with its activities and research dependent on government and institutional funding. She views psychologists as pawns in a larger industrial and economic game that manufactures dependent, conforming and disciplined members of the general public. Dineen adds that the profession of psychology on occasions has subverted truth into 'egocentric possessions' (p. 255) and manufactured truths to expand their activities and profits. Pilgrim (1997) has described similar functions as professional dominance that flows from social enclosure. Professionals exercise dominance over others in three ways. First, they hold power over clients by their use of specialised knowledge rendering others ignorant, dependent, vulnerable and insecure. Second, professionals hold power over new recruits via selection and hierarchy of decisions. Third, professionals seek dominant relationships over other professionals working with the same group of people.

I have no doubt that most of us working in services for people experiencing extreme turmoil are well meaning and that we apply ourselves with the best of intentions. We are often working in stressful situations guided by conventional structures and practice based on what seemingly is the most available knowledge to us. It is the basis of such knowledge and this context that I am questioning as limited in its helpfulness. Put simply, we are barking up the wrong tree. We must move away from a framework premised on a positivist reductionism, and currently this is what the NICE evidence for practice is founded on, with its advocacy of the random controlled trial as the gold standard of evidence. Psychiatry and clinical psychology services must replace the current limited epidemiological constraint that rarely considers factors beyond the individual with a heuristic exploratory enquiry. The latter recognises the salience of historical, social and material contexts and ultimately contributes towards a more meaningful and helpful understanding of human despair.

CRITICAL REALIST FRAMEWORK

There is much to learn from a critical realist framework. As human beings, I believe we are the embodiment of experiences that are founded on social and materialist histories. This is a separate topic in itself and I don't want to move too far away from the focus of the chapter. A social-materialist and critical-realist view acknowledges that individual development occurs within a social, economic and political context. Pilgrim and Bentall, (1999) refer to critical realism when attempting to understand scientific and technical concepts. They suggest that such concepts should be examined in the context of the social and historical conditions which allowed them to emerge and that this is indispensable. The theories and methods we adopt in the pursuit of knowledge are shaped by social forces and inevitably informed by interests and values. Such a position sits between (a) medical naturalism and (b) unending relativism of social constructionism. Cromby and Nightingale (1999), in making a case for critical realism, highlight the following: the importance of the influence of embodied factors and personal-social histories; the inherent constraints that shape our social constructions; and the power of institutions and governments. They draw on the problematic and limited nature of discourse when it is not embedded in the material world. They conclude:

> [F]rom a realist perspective, our social constructions are always already mediated in and through our embodied nature, the materiality of the world and pre-existing matrices of social and institutional power. (p. 209)

The task for a more transparent psychological practice then is to clarify the forces that impinge on our functioning. These forces are both social and material. They are something we are immersed in and continually moulded by their pressures. A thorough scientific search for all factors that affect human behaviour could not condone omitting such influences. It sometimes appears that the services we work in are determined to simply consider factors that are in some way part of the individual. Our task is to question the taken-for-granted sense of objectivity which in reality, at best, minimises and, at worst, ignores other professional and political influences on social injustices. Dineen (1999) documents the vested interests within the profession of psychology that flagrantly promote their own professional interests and values. Seider, Davis and Gardner (2007) recognise the cut-throat nature of the professional environment and the readiness of aspiring psychology professionals to cut corners and compromise their ethical moorings in order to compete with their peers. Prilleltensky and Nelson (2002) note the limitations of a psychology profession that fails to acknowledge its own position of power particularly in exerting influence on systems that maintain a dominant knowledge base.

Critical and liberationist social psychology of Latin America suggests that one cannot be impartial in the face of injustice (Burton, 2004; Jimenez-Dominguez, 2005). Drawing upon the work of Ignacio Martin-Baro, the ongoing importance of de-ideologisation is noted as core in the critical nature of scientific commitment. This would be the equivalent of objectivity, and it consists of dismantling the justifications that mask historical reality and removing the rationalisations of everyday social life. This would involve:

> bringing to the task of psychology a clear consciousness of its political repercussions, as well as bringing a consciousness of the psychological dimensions to the task of politics. We would say that it means creating a political consciousness for psychology and devising a psychology for political consciousness. (Jimenez-Dominguez, 2005: 68)

When considering the roles and functions of social and political contexts we need to acknowledge issues of power, interests and values. How can we develop more accountability and work towards a sense of transparency? In essence, how do we uncover a fuller explanation that may contribute to a real sense of what it is to experience the depths of despair? I realise, in calling for a truth that acknowledges the vested interests of any scientific enquiry I am opening up a can of philosophical worms. Whilst it is not the purpose of this chapter to consider these issues at length, I would like to briefly refer to sources that have called for similar truths in different contexts. C. Wright Mills (2000) calls for a return to the sociological imagination that goes beyond Western bureaucratised science that uses rationality to pursue its own end, to maintain power by exerting functions of coercion, authority and manipulation. He says:

> [R]ationally organised social arrangements are not necessarily a means of increased freedom for the individual or for society. In fact, often they are a means of tyranny and manipulation, a means of expropriating the very chance to reason, the very capacity to act as a free man. (p. 169)

The novelist Kurt Vonnegut (1998) calls for us to respect our human awareness or soul that stretches across this world, in doing so moving out of the ever-expanding, seemingly never-ending pursuit of material and self-centred needs. Calling for more ordinariness, Vonnegut describes the challenge to each of us to behave decently in an indecent society. Mary Boyle (2006), calls upon psychologists to at least head towards speaking truths about ourselves or at least to comment on the truths we are still not speaking. She adds, that in spite of strong evidence about the importance of people's relationships and social circumstances in the development, maintenance and expression of emotional and behavioural problems, we continue to privilege theories which locate problems inside people's heads. Referring to the profession of clinical psychology, David Smail (2002) comments that the developments and trends of psychology, what he describes as the vagaries of fashion, have nothing to do with scientific progress—there is no sign of an emergent unifying paradigm. Smail continues, the positioning of the profession seems in fact to have been much more about our attempts to situate ourselves as advantageously as possible within the structures of power that determine the profession's interests. Smail, therefore, calls for the theories and practices of clinical psychology to be founded on an authority that is independent of the profession's interests.

It would seem then that the structures and functions of power not only maintain order to an existing system but simultaneously promote the vested interests of professional groups that occupy positions of privilege. Those in privileged positions remain so through retention of a discourse that promotes their opinions whilst at the same time quietening the voices of the marginalised. This is achieved by closing down public spaces that would otherwise enable the articulation of views other than those of the current incumbents of power (Fanon, 1986; Foucault, 1989; Rose, 1999). Taiwo Afuape (2006) looks at the subjugated voices across the world. She talks of the quietened majority voices of Africa, Asia, Far and Middle East and Latin America, quietened by the minority yet imperialist and oppressive dominance of Western psychology. She shows how subjugating voices from the majority world leads to an incomplete understanding of human beings based on the insights of dominant voices from the minority of the world. She calls for an interconnected balance of community and spirit and emphasises the importance of otherness and mutuality as opposed to the

> Western world's aggressive cultural imperialism and fanatical expansionism which requires the continuous search for new lands, people and objects to conquer. (p. 244)

The particular questions that we ask about our circumstances govern the answers that we elicit. What would the services we work in look like if we were less concerned with the existing dominant order of psychiatry and clinical psychology and instead opened up spaces for consideration of what Afuape calls otherness and mutuality? Smail (2002: 10), with regard to the concepts of power and interest, suggests:

> if ever we are to get at least a conceptual grip on those pervasive and intractable aspects of human suffering that are our own making, we are going to have to struggle with the ways in which power and interest shape our lives as well as the structures of meaning that filter our understanding of our plight ... The task is to develop a language that *articulates* our relations to reality as accurately as possible.

ARTICULATING A QUESTIONING PSYCHOLOGY

So what to do about it? How to set about such articulation? Perhaps a starting point would be to unpick some of the needlework that has woven together the threads of power, interests and values into a selective tapestry that is depicted as the accepted cloth of conventional wisdom and knowledge. We must not only acknowledge but start to address the imbalance of particular privileged theories that reside over marginalised or silenced accounts of our understanding of health. I would like to consider, in the first instance, the role, functions and position of the health service.

Within existing mental health services, Prilleltensky (1997) contends the discourse and power structures maintain a dominant order that promote concepts of care, health and compassion, which to some extent ameliorates personal discomfort and distress. However, both Prilleltensky (1997) and Kagan and Burton (2001) suggest that a transformational process of change is required which includes not only care, health and compassion but also, social justice, self-determination and equality. The dominant discourse within psychiatry and clinical psychology is structured around concepts and values that are familiar to the professions in practice; it is a discourse that essentially describes pathologies of the individual. In this instance this is the inner, or status quo, the accepted wisdom. Whilst we may have witnessed some developments in recent years that appear to influence the centre, or inner position, nonetheless, the inner view remains largely cautious and preserves the status quo. For example, people with experiences of using mental health services have been encouraged to become more involved in expressing their views and influencing the future of such services, however, to date, such influences appear to have made little if any impact (Pilgrim & Waldron, 2002; Diamond et al, 2003). It almost seems as though any dissent by people with experiences of using mental health services has been absorbed within the inner structures of the existing order. The values and interests of those representing the inner, or the status quo, almost seem incapable of enabling further dissent that might lead to significant changes to the existing order.

What would it look like both conceptually and practically to move from a position within the centre of the dominant order, that is, the inner, along a spectrum to a position that embraced values beyond the existing accepted knowledge base. Figure 1 is adapted from Holland (1992) and is a spatial representation using axes of regulation (status quo) and radical change set against different positions within the established order, within and beyond the conventions of the day. I accept this is contentious; I am simply keen to explore where, if at all, change can come about and also where the most fruitful grounds for the seeds of change and development are located.

What might the dotted line in Figure 1 look like? Is it possible to describe such a position? What might it include? This chapter has called for greater transparency within psychiatry and clinical psychology services about our practice. Could such values and position offer anything towards a more legitimate authority, perhaps towards a greater transparency of our work?

FUNCTION
RADICAL CHANGE

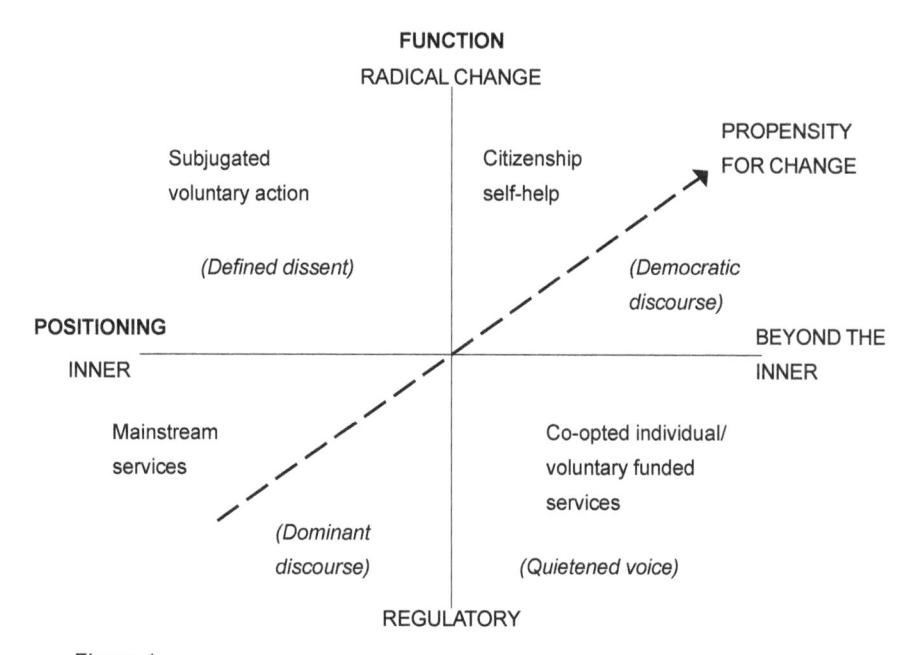

		PROPENSITY FOR CHANGE
Subjugated voluntary action	Citizenship self-help	
(Defined dissent)	*(Democratic discourse)*	

POSITIONING _____ BEYOND THE
INNER   INNER

Mainstream services	Co-opted individual/ voluntary funded services
(Dominant discourse)	*(Quietened voice)*

REGULATORY

Figure 1.

The current establishment of psychiatry and clinical psychology, something I am referring to as the inner values position, tend to work towards the values, functions and interests that are: individual, normative, personal/professional, benignly benevolent, defined coalescent discourse, by this I mean an agreement on what is accepted as discourse by the existing services and based on notions of independence and free-will (see Table 1). I am suggesting services would be more meaningful and informative if they embraced values, functions and interests that included: social, material and environmental factors, were diverse and inclusive in their functions, promoted interests that were not only personal and professional but also societal. Such a position would also promote equality and have an emancipatory role, accommodate elaborated dissent, a dissent that would not immediately be subjugated in to the dominant order. This position would also look beyond the aspiration of independence to an interdependence and political awareness of social structures that influence our well-being. Ultimately, by moving away from a preoccupation with the present inner dominant order we would move away from the contemporary obsession with the self and open up space to acknowledge the importance of the relational qualities of linking with others that significantly affect our health. The tentative ideas expressed in Table 1 are influenced by community and critical psychology and have much in common with the comparisons Bostock (1998a) makes between clinical psychology and community psychology, and also the importance recognised by Prilleltensky and Nelson (2002) that well-being is not merely a matter of attending to the self but equally to relational and societal contexts.

Working towards greater transparency in services requires acknowledging the balance of dissension with conformity and the importance of recognising our own position, power and agenda when attempting to work critically. It is important to consider ways of working towards a transparency that embraces sharing with, rather than doing to, others, uses ordinary language rather than specialist language, works with humility and modesty rather than expertise, is willing to share information and learn from others and acknowledges the importance of unfamiliarity and uncertainty. Many of these values are advocated by community psychology.

Table 1

	Existing order—services (Inner)	Beyond established order
Focus	Individual	Social, material and environmental
Functions	Normative and invited	Diverse and inclusive
Interests	Personal and professional	Personal, professional and societal
Values	Benign benevolence	Equality promoting and emancipatory
Discourse	Defined coalescence	Elaborated dissent
Aspirations	Independence and free will	Interdependence and poltical awareness
Knowledge	Self	Relational

TOWARDS A MORE TRANSPARENT PSYCHOLOGICAL PRACTICE

Bostock and Diamond (2005) suggest community psychology broadens our focus from individual and reactive interventions and creates opportunities to voice the links between social circumstances and psychological well-being. Community psychology reminds us of our limitations as psychological therapists and advocates for social change and working collaboratively with others. Thus future community and clinical psychology services need to share and learn from others, particularly disempowered groups and communities; understand the operation of power; use ordinary language that embraces tolerance, modesty and humility; and work energetically and creatively with uncertainty, and potentially conflicting interests.

The salient principles of community psychology are:

- Working with communities as well as individuals. That is, groups that share common interests. Build alliances with marginalised groups. A recognition that peer support can be mutually benefiting and an effective means to change.
- Encouraging collaborative and participative involvement of both individuals and communities. Such involvement may contribute to developing both practical activities as well as new knowledge.

- An approach that seeks to develop people's strengths rather than focus on concepts such as diagnoses or categorising symptoms.

- Acknowledging the importance of primary influences such as housing, income, social circumstances as well as histories on well-being.

- Emphasising prevention rather than reaction or treatment. This may take the form of education, facilitating social support, influencing public policy.

- A commitment to devolve professional power and to work in the interests of sharing control and decision-making.

- Engaging in action to address and overcome pathology within service systems and society.

- Recognition of social injustices. Aim to affect social change in a broad context. Active in influencing social policy that facilitates the empowerment of disadvantaged and disenfranchised people.

Such considerations summarise an orientation and value position that informs practice. Rather than representing a technique or specific intervention, community psychology is built around a framework of principles and its practice may look different and relatively unique to each setting. Community psychology is committed to working towards greater social equality and embraces particular values such as inclusion, justice, freedom and respect. There are many examples of community psychology in practice and, whilst it is not the remit of this chapter to consider them in detail, these include, housing environments (Edge, Stewart & Kagan, 2004; Kagan, 2007), debt and poverty (Bostock, 2004), people who use mental health services and their involvement (Diamond et al, 2003), women's health (Holland, 1992) employment and local groups (Fryer, 1990, 1992), and research (Serrano-Garcia, 1990).

The importance of opening up space and opportunities for hitherto quietened voices was demonstrated over the past twenty years by developments involving people who hear voices (Downs, 2005). The Hearing Voices Network demonstrated how other perspectives than those represented by the establishment can successfully challenge the dominant existing order of psychiatry. This work started in the late 1980s when the majority of psychiatric training texts simply referred to hearing voices as symptoms of illness best treated by medication, and those hearing voices were to be encouraged to distract and discourage any efforts to engage with voices. Any dissenting voice from the established order of psychiatry was either minimised or ignored. Any attempts to consider alternative concepts tended to create anxiety amongst staff. Consequently staff were apprehensive about developing dialogues with people hearing voices. Over time and with perseverance and pressures from the self-help networks, particularly the Hearing Voices Network (Downs, 2005) there has been some acceptance of the importance of people's own experiences in coping with the distress they experience. Some 15 years later, open dialogue between voice hearer, voices and staff is shown to be essential in supporting people who hear voices to cope with the distress they experience. For an example of this work see Diamond (1998). There are many accounts of alternative explanations for distress that go beyond the present rather limited psychiatric concepts of distress (Romme & Escher, 2000; Coleman, 2004; Harper, 2004). Psychiatry must acknowledge its current limitations and be willing to open up opportunities to learn from others. To do this psychiatry must suspend if not relinquish some of its strongly held beliefs, create space for dissension and afford more respect to other accounts.

Another area where I believe we are all too complicit in acceding to the conventions of the day is in the practice of individual psychological help. We have chosen selectively to base our professional endeavours, such as counselling and psychotherapy, on particular foundations that in my view are misguided in promoting the potency of the individual over social and material considerations. This is nothing new; people have been raising similar concerns for quite some time, (Lomas, 1987; Dineen, 1999; Masson, 1990; Smail, 2001; Epstein, 2006). However, it would appear that the current preoccupation with, for example, cognitive behaviour therapy (CBT) has much deeper political ramifications and is no longer simply a benign philanthropic endeavour that may be considered a naïve shot at helping people in distress. Witness the purportedly quick-fix CBT approach advocated by Lord Layard (2006) as a means of reducing income capacity benefit payments. Such proposals are part of Layard's whole-hearted yet ill-informed and misguided notion of the everyday pursuit of happiness. Again here is an example of services attributing distress to the supposed limitations and faults of the individual by proposing intrapersonal faulty or dysfunctional cognitive schemata.

A questioning psychology would steer away from the focus on intrapersonal faults and limitations, in preference to opening up space for consideration of an environmental, strengths-based framework. This would encourage personal value and meaningful connections, where possible, to social contexts. Perhaps this is where some of the values, interests and functions described as beyond the established order in Table 1 may inform us. There are a number of examples of practice where people experiencing enduring distress and often living in extremely disruptive circumstances are receiving help and support in ways that go beyond traditional one-to-one therapy, (Knight, 2005; May, 2006). I have no doubt that psychological therapies based on a confidential one-to-one approach will continue, why shouldn't they? After all we would not be human if we did not seek the comforting company of others. I would be disingenuous not to acknowledge that this is a key part of my work. Nonetheless, I think it would be helpful to move away from the notion of individual responsibility that can so easily slide into culpability; we should also express more realism and caution over our prospects and abilities to be both architect and engineer of whatever outlook and quality of life we may desire.

Having expressed reservations and limitations about the efficacy of psychotherapy, I would argue for a form of psychological help that retains elements of emotional, social and practical help; a framework that encourages clarification through curiosity, comfort through reassurance, and strives literally and metaphorically towards a connectedness through personal, social and material resources, ultimately to gain, whenever possible, some sense of increased influence in our lives. Figure 2 shows the importance of three areas in therapeutic support: being taken seriously, doing and acting together, and supportive conversations. Together, I suggest they form what is typically referred to as therapeutic support. These areas do not exist within the vacuum of the therapy clinic, rather they are always immersed in the 'impress of power' (Smail, 2005).

I sometimes wonder whether psychotherapists are sufficiently mindful of the influence of contexts and settings that are imposed upon people they seek to help (Bostock, 1998b; Meltzer et al, 2000). Social and material contexts are inextricably linked with well-being. Despite our best efforts at meaningful conversations and encouragement, such living environments are highly unlikely to change for most people. It would seem that the essential functions and underlying qualities of psychological help are comforting and clarifying (Smail, 2001). Supportive and therapeutic conversations are, amongst other things, shared understandings with some agreements between workers and clients that provide helpful explanations of situations clients find themselves in. They guide and inform the aims and goals for practical, social and psychological work between workers and clients: they also start from the very first point of meeting one another and remain throughout all contacts ranging from the practical to how a person is feeling. Therapeutic conversations are, whenever possible, ultimately about supporting someone to make a little more sense of their situation and develop more meaning and purpose in their life by linking in some way with others.

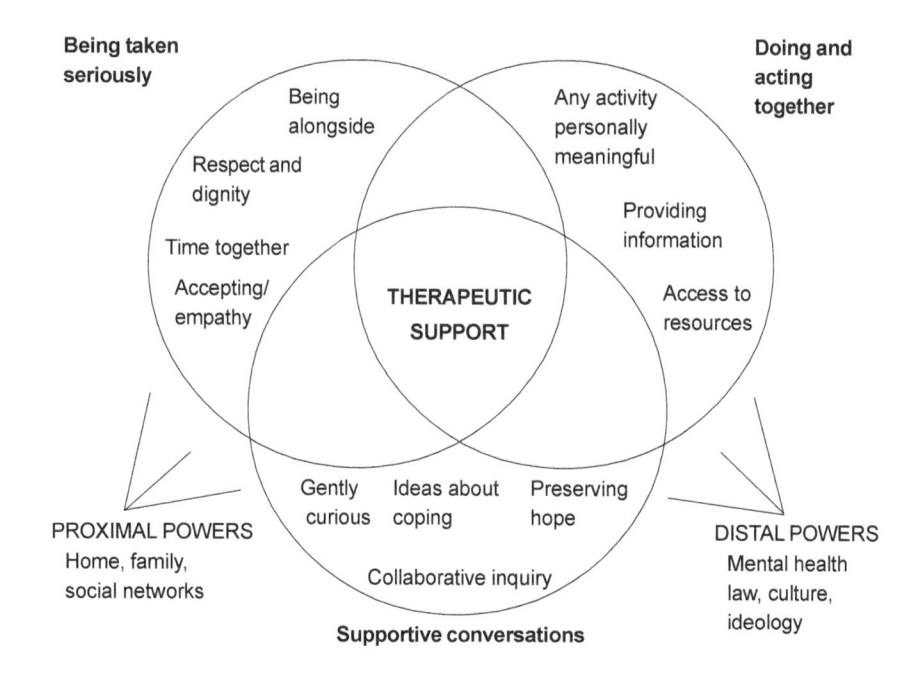

Figure 2. Therapeutic Engagement in Mental Health Services

Supportive and therapeutic conversations are based on relationships that have some trust and mutual respect. Only when these values are established is it really possible to work alongside clients and gently enquire. Only by remaining respectful of much of the sense that clients make of their worlds are workers able to keep a sensitive interest in and a hopeful curiosity about client's experiences. As therapeutic relationships develop, workers are able to weave what they have learnt from clients with their knowledge and practice into shared understandings that guide them when offering support. As workers listen and learn from clients, in turn they are able to reflect the sense they are making of situations. Such understandings should be tentatively shared with clients and a reciprocal process of learning and sharing allows a unique 'best fit' frame of reference to evolve. This, coupled with a focus on supporting people to connect with whatever resources that may be available to them, may assist a person to retrieve or possibly develop connections with others. By resources I am referring to such areas in our lives that are described by Hagan and Smail in power mapping (1997a, b); these include home and family life, social life, personal resources and material resources. Therefore, as workers in psychiatry and clinical psychology, we should at least acknowledge and if at all possible support people to gain access to whatever resources may be humanly possible; I accept that so often it may not be possible. More often than not, such opportunities are extremely limited and often non-existent. In such circumstances, we still have a role in acknowledging the trapped situation people find themselves in. It may be helpful to some degree to clarify through a process of elaboration why we may feel as we do, but does such awareness necessarily lead to change? The literature on psychotherapies tends to obfuscate what happens beyond clarification. Some psychotherapy aims to help clients achieve 'insight', although the term itself is unclear; once this is gained it is claimed that improvements in clients' lives are likely to come about. I am less convinced by this argument, preferring to consider that it is access to, or more importantly, the *lack* of access to resources that is crucial to any likelihood of positive changes.

I do not want to negate the role of developing a sense of relatedness or being together (see Figure 2) which, hopefully, should occur in any psychologically supportive relationship. This, I believe is what is behind the supportive evidence for non-specific factors in therapy, such as trust, respect, consent and negotiated agreement on the nature of discussions and outcomes. Of course a sense of closeness which I have described as 'being together' is very important; it is hard to imagine a setting where potentially one person is asked the most intimate of questions without a sense of trust and closeness. However, sometimes, I think this sense of trust, respect and confiding can be overoptimistically understood as a marker of significant life changes. This, I believe, is unfortunate although very understandable in a system that places such credence on the perceived potential power of the individual.

In conclusion, a critical or questioning psychology is much more than simply dismissing the conventions of the day. It encourages dialogue between conformity and dissension and opens up constructive space to elaborate our current understandings of, in this instance, human distress. Critical constructive theory and practice invites us to acknowledge our own agenda and position of power, share with others as opposed to do to others, using ordinary rather than specialist language, embracing humility and modesty and acknowledging the importance of unfamiliarity and uncertainty. With foundations based on mutual respect and dignity along with cornerstones of integrity, critical constructive theory and practice endeavours to look out for, and whenever possible, salvage something from the desolation and despair experienced by many people.

REFERENCES

Afuape, T (2006) Subjugating nature and 'the other': Deconstructing dominant themes in minority world culture and their implications for Western psychology. *Journal of Critical Psychology, Counselling and Psychotherapy,* 6 (4), 238–55.
Bostock, J (1998a) From clinic to community: Generating social validity in clinical psychology. *Clinical Psychology Forum,* 121, 2–6.
Bostock, J (1998b) Developing coherence in community and clinical psychology: The integration of idealism and pragmatism. *Journal of Community & Applied Social Psychology,* 8, 1–9.
Bostock, J (2004) Addressing poverty and exploitation: Challenges for psychology. *Clinical Psychology,* 38, 23–7.
Bostock, J & Diamond, R (2005) The value of community psychology: Critical reflections from the NHS. *Clinical Psychology Forum,* 153, 22–5.
Boyle, M (2006) Speaking the truth about ourselves. *Clinical Psychology Forum,* 168, 4–6.
Burton, M (2004) Viva Nacho! Liberating psychology in Latin America. *The Psychologist, 17* (10), 584–7.
Charlton, B (2000) The new management of scientific knowledge in medicine: A change of direction with profound implications. In A Miles, JR Hampton & B Hurwitz (Eds) *NICE, CHI and the NHS Reforms: Enabling excellence or imposing control?* (pp 13–31). London: Aesculapius Medical Press.
Coleman, R (2004) *Recovery: An alien concept* (2nd edn). Dundee: P&P Press.
Cromby, J & Nightingale, D (Eds) (1999) *Social Constructionist Psychology: A critical analysis of theory and practice.* Buckingham: Open University Press.
Diamond, R (1998) Stepping outside and not knowing: Community psychology and enduring mental health problems. *Clinical Psychology Forum,* 12, 40–2.
Diamond, R (2004) Expert-tease: The rise and rise of psychology. *Journal of Critical psychology, Counselling and Psychotherapy,* 4 (4), 242–6.
Diamond, R, Parkin, G, Morris, K, Bettinis, J & Bettesworth, C (2003) User involvement: Substance or spin? *Journal of Mental Health,* 12 (6), 613–26.
Dineen, T (1999) *Manufacturing Victims: What the psychology industry is doing to people.* London: Constable.
Double, D (Ed) (2006) *Critical Psychiatry: The limits of madness.* Basingstoke: Palgrave Macmillan.
Downs, J (2005) *Coping with Voices and Visions.* Manchester: Hearing Voices Network.
Edge, I, Stewart, A & Kagan, C (2004) Living poverty: Surviving on the edge. *Clinical Psychology,* 38, 28–31.
Epstein, WM (2006) *Psychotherapy as Religion: The civil divine in America.* Reno, NV: University of Nevada Press.
Fanon, F (1986) *Black Skin, White Masks.* London: Pluto Press.
Foucault, M (1989) *The Birth of the Clinic.* Abingdon: Routledge.
Fryer, D (1990) The mental health consequences of unemployment: Towards a social psychological concept of poverty. *British Journal of Clinical and Social Psychiatry,* 7 (4), 164–76.

Fryer, D (1992) Signed on at the 'beroo': Mental health and unemployment in Scotland. *The Psychologist, 5,* 539–42.
Hagan, T & Smail, D (1997a) Power-mapping: I. Background and basic methodology. *Journal of Community and Applied Social Psychology, 7,* 257–67.
Hagan, T & Smail, D (1997b) Power-mapping: II. Practical application: the example of child sexual abuse. *Journal of Community and Applied Social Psychology, 7,* 269–84.
Harper, D (2004) Delusions and discourse: Moving beyond the constraints of the modernist paradigm. *Philosophy, Psychiatry, & Psychology, 11* (1), 55–64.
Holland, S (1992) From social abuse to social action: A neighbourhood psychotherapy and social action project for women. *Changes, 10* (2), 146–53.
Jimenez-Dominguez, BH (2005) The critical and liberationist social psychology of Ignacio Martin-Baro: An objection to objectivism. *Journal of Critical Psychology, Counselling and Psychotherapy 5* (2), 63–9.
Johnstone, L (2000) *Users & Abusers of Psychiatry: A critical look at traditional psychiatric practice* (2nd edn). London: Routledge.
Kagan, C (2007) Working at the edge: Making use of psychological resources through collaboration. *The Psychologist, 20* (4), 224–7.
Kagan, C & Burton, M (2001) Critical community psychology praxis for the 21st century. Paper presented to British Psychological Society conference, Glasgow, March.
Knight, T (2005) You'd better believe it: Accepting and working within the client's own reality. *Clinical Psychology Forum, 155,* 38–42.
Layard, R (2006) *Happiness: Lessons from a new science.* London: Penguin.
Lomas, P (1987) *The Limits of Interpretation: What's wrong with psychoanalysis.* London: Penguin.
Lynch, T (2006) Understanding psychiatry's resistance to change. In D Double (Ed) *Critical Psychiatry: The limits of madness* (pp 99–113). Basingstoke: Palgrave Macmillan.
Masson, J (1990) *Against Therapy.* London: Fontana.
May, R (2006) Resisting the diagnostic gaze. *Journal of Critical Psychology, Counselling and Psychotherapy, 6* (3), 155–8.
Meltzer, H, Singleton, N, Lee, A, Bebbington, P, Brugha, T & Jenkins, R (2000) *The Social and Economic Circumstances of Adults with Mental Disorders.* London: National Statistics Office.
Moloney, P (2006) The trouble with psychotherapy. *Clinical Psychology Forum, 162,* 29–33.
Moncrieff, J (2006) The politics of psychiatric drug treatment. In D Double (Ed) *Critical Psychiatry: The limits of madness* (pp 115–32). Basingstoke: Palgrave Macmillan.
Pilgrim, D (1997) *Psychotherapy and Society.* London: Sage.
Pilgrim, D & Bentall, R (1999) The medicalisation of misery: A critical realist analysis of the concept of depression. *Journal of Mental Health, 8* (3), 261–74.
Pilgrim, D & Waldron, L (2002) Use involvement in mental health services development: How far can it go? *Journal of Mental Health, 7* (1), 95–104.
Prilleltensky, I (1997) Community psychology: Reclaiming social justice. In D Fox & I Prilleltensky (Eds) *Critical Psychology: An introduction* (pp 166–84). London: Sage.
Prilleltensky, I & Nelson, G (2002) *Doing Psychology Critically: Making a difference in diverse settings.* Basingstoke: Palgrave Macmillan.
Read, J & Reynolds, J (Eds) (1996) *Speaking our Minds: An anthology.* Basingstoke: Macmillan.
Rogers, A & Pilgrim, D (2003) *Mental Health Inequality.* Basingstoke: Palgrave Macmillan.
Romme, M & Escher, S (2000) *Making Sense of Voices.* London: Mind Publications.
Rose, N (1999) *Governing the Soul: The shaping of the private self* (2nd edn). London Free Association Books.

Seider, S, Davis, K & Gardner, H (2007) Good work in psychology. *The Psychologist, 20* (11), 672–6.
Serrano-Garcia, I (1990) Implementing research: Putting our values to work. In P Tolan, C Keys, F Chertok & L Jason (Eds) *Researching Community Psychology: Issues of theory and methods* (pp 171–82). New York: American Psychological Association.
Smail, D (2001) *The Nature of Unhappiness.* London: Robinson.
Smail, D (2002) Psychology and power: Understanding human action. *Journal of Critical Psychology, Counselling and Psychotherapy, 2,* 1–10.
Smail, D (2005) *Power, Interest and Psychology.* Ross-on-Wye: PCCS Books.
Timimi, S (2006) Critical child psychiatry. In D Double (Ed) *Critical Psychiatry: The limits of madness* (pp 189–206). Basingstoke: Palgrave Macmillan.
Vonnegut, K (1998) *Timequake.* London: Vintage.
Wallcraft, J & Michaelson, J (2001) Developing a survivor discourse to replace the 'psychopathology' of breakdown and crisis. In C Newnes, G Holmes & C Dunn (Eds) *This is Madness Too: Critical perspectives on mental health services* (pp 177–90). Ross-on-Wye: PCCS Books.
Wright Mills, C (2000) *The Sociological Imagination.* New York: Oxford University Press.

Acknowledgements
I would like to thank Jan Bostock and David Smail for their helpful comments on this chapter.

CHAPTER 13

CLINICAL PSYCHOLOGY AND TRUTH*

DAVID SMAIL

Forty-odd years ago I was an enthusiastic researcher into and advocate of the therapeutic community movement in psychiatry. For someone who started his career in a large Victorian mental hospital in Surrey, the writings of psychiatrists such as Denis Martin (e.g. Martin, 1962) and Maxwell Jones (e.g. Jones, 1952) (who knows of them now?) promised a positive liberation from the medical straitjacket that enclosed people, metaphorically if not literally. Around the same time, research started to appear that lent real support to the hypothesis that social (particularly, of course, family) background was crucial to an understanding of so-called illnesses such as 'schizophrenia' (e.g. Jackson, 1960; Lidz et al, 1965; Scott & Ashworth, 1965).

I read R.D. Laing's early books with real excitement, and I heard him speak in the early sixties: serious, intelligent, brave, then and now the foremost among the very few truly creative and intellectually compelling voices of British psychiatry. Both in relation to 'diagnosis' and 'treatment', freedom was in the air. Not just mindless rebellion, but considered, reasoned, and, to an encouraging extent, empirically supported objections to the stuffy, authoritarian dogmas of conventional psychiatry. There were even times in the seventies when orthodox psychiatry seemed to be on the back foot—I can remember junior psychiatrists worrying that they would be out of a job sooner rather than later if they didn't find alternatives to the biomedical model.

So what happened? More or less coincident with the Thatcher/Reagan counter-revolution and the re-emergence of the Right, Mental Illness came back with a vengeance, supported by a biologism as dogmatic as it had ever been earlier in the century. Quietly forgetting its doubtful past in the Eugenics movement, genetics once again took centre-stage, confidently claiming the support of new technology. Laing's perspective was dismissed on the basis of his later descent into celebrity and alcoholism, and, with one or two somewhat tepid exceptions, research into the social background of madness was abandoned for fear of 'blaming' parents.

In order to support psychiatric pretensions, and no doubt cognisant of the requirements of the pharmaceutical industry, that farcical instrument, the *Diagnostic and Statistical Manual of Mental Disorders* was developed in a series of editions each more bizarre than the last.

I can't speak for the physical sciences and the technologies they engender—presumably we all have an interest in their flourishing, and hence, to some extent at least, leave them to get on with it—but in the social sciences and indeed the rest of the

*This is a slightly expanded version of a talk given at the University of East London in September 2007, on the occasion of Professor Mary Boyle's retirement.

culture, empirically based critical reason—what one takes to be the very basis of science—all but disappeared in the last quarter of the twentieth century. Indeed, words like 'empirical' and 'reason' came under attack at the highest intellectual levels.

Magic and make-believe re-emerge as respectable methods of structuring social relations. Fundamentalist religions enjoy a surprising revival and political reality comes to be determined by spin. 'Complementary' medicine establishes its place in the NHS with royal endorsement. In psychology, the constraining rule of positivist behaviourism is replaced seemingly overnight by a kind of neo-philosophical idealism (fitted loosely under the umbrella of 'postmodernism') that warrants a comfortable relativism. Cognitions and discourses replace empirical reality and psychoanalysis is raised from the almost-dead to take its place alongside a range of therapeutic brands from which the consumer can make an uncritical choice.

All these events are of course not unrelated. Following an irksome banishment to the wings after two devastating World Wars, the triumphant re-establishment of capitalist economic structures and institutions reverberates throughout the world and penetrates just about every aspect of social relations. For all we therapist clinicians waffle about 'change', it is practical women and men of the world who, like Margaret Thatcher, really know how to bring it about. Offer a few juicy carrots and you will bring the worst out of the greedy and ambitious; wave a big, menacing stick (like threatening their livelihoods) and you will have just about everyone else jumping smartly into line.

Did heads of NHS departments refuse to implement the new business strategies that made a mockery of all they stood for? No, they queued up to become managers. Did the University vice-chancellors and pro-vice-chancellors defend academic freedom and independence; did they speak out for 'Reason and Right' as, in the face of fascist oppression years before, had Miguel de Unamuno, the Rector of Salamanca University?[1] No, they formed committees to decide how to institute redundancies, cut courses and sell their degrees abroad. Did ordinary men and women rise up against the economic and disciplinary practices that threatened their jobs, undermined their solidarity and stole their pensions? No, they blamed themselves and looked for a therapist.

The Business ideology that corporate capitalism gives rise to has no use for the pursuit of truth; it consists rather of a crude pragmatism: what's right and good is what works ('what works' in this context usually of course meaning 'what makes money'). This ideology has become so embedded in the culture now that it's become difficult to think outside it, even for those who want to. Psychological therapists, for example, often find it quite hard to entertain the idea that a given approach or technique could be wrong—misleading, mistaken, nonsensical even—if it 'works', in the sense, perhaps, of changing people in some way. But changing and controlling people is easy. You can do

---

1. Unamuno in a confrontation with fascist General Milan-Astray at the University of Salamanca on October 12, 1936: 'At times to be silent is to lie. You will win because you have enough brute force. But you will not convince. For to convince you need to persuade. And in order to persuade you would need what you lack: Reason and Right.' Milan-Astray shouted in reply, *'Death to intelligence! And long live Death!'* whereupon he drove the elderly Unamuno out of the university at gunpoint. Unamuno consequently suffered a heart attack and was dead within a week. http://www.rjgeib.com/heroes/unamuno/unamuno.html

it in all sorts of ways: put a gun in their backs, doctor the water supply, put them out of a job, stupefy them with consumerist junk and celebrity claptrap, and so on. The Business mind is an uncomplicated one; impatient with the kind of critical cavilling it sees as typical of intellectuals and dismissive of the social structures and institutions that had evolved (however imperfectly) to nurture the pursuit of truth.

What we need, according to the Business view, is not to find the truth, but to achieve targets and solve problems. Boil things down to their essentials; establish appropriate divisions of labour such that what anyone does accords with management aims; isolate the active ingredients of intellectual and professional enquiry; establish the 'evidence base'; amalgamate and homogenise knowledge so that its essence can be extracted (as with 'meta-analyses') and put to work towards achievement of the targets or solution of the problems.

This kind of mechanised approach to problem solution has nothing to do with trying to discover the reasons for things. Its justification usually is the maximisation of profit. A good test of whether something works is whether it pays off. Whether or not it's true is not just uninteresting, it's irrelevant. If enough people say they feel better after six sessions of 'cognitive re-structuring', that's good enough; who cares whether 'cognitive re-structuring' makes any sense at all as an hypothetical entity?

Reason has no place in this debased form of neo-pragmatism, and applied social disciplines such as psychology become entirely detached from the passionate need to locate our place within the world and explicate our relations to it, which characterises scientific enquiry. Indeed, we find philosophies flourishing in which there *is* no reality independent of ourselves: if we cock an ear to the universe we hear only our own discourse.

Things have reached such a pass in this respect that it is now possible for a 'Principal Lecturer in Psychology and Mental Health' to express in a relatively serious publication views such as the following (Forshaw, 2007):

> My postmodern, poststructuralist method of choice would probably be entirely akin to a form of loose literary criticism. Read, think, posit. Tag on a theoretical approach if you will. Take an atheoretical stance of you wish ... Spend weeks if it suits you, spend minutes if you prefer. The conclusion of your research will be the same: a set of interpretations and some suggestions as to what might be. Just try to resist the temptation to think that you are solving something. None of us are. Pushing a sealed treasure chest around the floor is not the same thing as picking the lock and opening it. Even if we could pick the lock, there is no guarantee that there is anything inside. (p. 479)

Here is a philosophy of 'anything goes' from which everything has gone: intellectual discipline and concern with reality of course, but also coherence, respect for meaning, lucidity, ordinary competence with words. All that is left, it seems, is the opportunity for absolutely anyone to exploit the market in any way they can dream up.

Scientific enquiry, the search for truth, can best—perhaps only—be carried out in an unusually protected environment where, in return for their concentrated effort, practitioners are accorded a kind of social patronage with as few strings attached as possible. Curiosity, creativity, intellectual ingenuity need to be given absolutely free play. And always and again the notions scientists may have about the world need to be tested against the stubborn reality that can gainsay them. There are all sorts—perhaps an infinity—of ways of doing this, and all attempts to define 'the scientific method' and tie scientists down to conforming to it, are likely to fail. But the ultimate criterion is always the same: is the hypothesis supported despite our best attempts to disprove it? Does it tell us something about the nature of the world *beyond* our own imaginings?

Scientific enquiry can only flourish if scientists are *trusted* to get on with it. Trust can of course be misplaced—the occasional rogue scientist may fabricate results, or perhaps just spend the day doing crosswords and sipping gin and tonic (I have personally encountered both kinds). That's just too bad. But one thing that's sure to kill off scientific enquiry altogether is the determination to control it managerially, to specify its outcomes and mechanise its procedures. In this kind of situation, untrammelled curiosity gives way to a very different kind of interest, and all the scientist's ingenuity goes into producing the kinds of results desired by those who control the budget. The requirement to *dis*prove gives way to the need to prove; doubts, for example, about the viability of schizophrenia as a disease entity are replaced by claims of its being 'incontrovertibly' a genetic disorder (and of course no proposition said to be incontrovertible can ever be a scientific one).

Instead of a scientific community collaborating openly and debating critically on publicly available data, there emerge *authorities* who pronounce on what can and cannot be considered to be the case; committees will be set up to ensure that only *authorised* ideas and procedures can be entertained, taught, and accredited. And what is authorised will be those ideas and procedures which further the interests of the controlling powers. It is precisely in this way that the critical interrogation of received ideas in the field of mental health gave way to, for example, the kind of assembly-line travesty of research results that NICE supplies for management to set its targets.

There was a time when clinical psychology claimed to be scientific. As is the case with so many social phenomena, this claim was, in my view anyway, shaped by the interest of a particular group—in this case of course clinical psychologists—in finding a role that would distinguish them from the competition—in this case of course psychiatrists, who had a total monopoly in the mental health sphere. This claim to being scientific, however, did mean that, when they were not skivvying for psychiatrists, many clinical psychologists could pursue more or less unhampered a research interest in various aspects of the causes, diagnosis and treatment of what was then thought of as mental illness. They could observe, read, and think critically, and test their observations and hypotheses, for the most part without undue interference from anyone higher up the hierarchy of power.

Secretly, though, this wasn't what most clinical psychologists *really* wanted to do. Being nice, well-meaning people who had probably drifted into the NHS mainly out of a desire to help people, what they really wanted to do was *treatment*, and since they had no medical qualifications, their best hope of getting involved in treatment was to find a way of making people better by talking to them. Since Freud had already thought of this, some clinical psychologists duly flirted with or became peripherally attached to psychodynamic approaches of one kind or another, but most leaped at the lifeline offered by the early proselytisers of behaviour therapy such as Hans Eysenck and Joseph Wolpe:

here, it seemed, was a treatment approach that not only did not require medical qualifications, but was 'scientific' to boot!

Of course, behaviour therapy wasn't scientific at all. Rather as cognitive behavioural therapy (CBT) does now, it claimed the *authority* of science by expressing its dogmas in what sounded like the discourse of scientific method, and then used that authority to browbeat doubters into silence. But most of us were probably happy enough to go along with the new behavioural dispensation anyway, since having our professional interests furthered was on the whole a lot more satisfying than having our doubts assuaged.

And so, with only a very little hesitation, we set ourselves on a course from which we have never looked back. We became, so to speak, professional healers, rapidly adopting whatever therapeutic rhetoric seemed most likely to convince our clients and our colleagues in the mental health field. Once the scientism of behaviour therapy became too obviously transparent to support a whole profession, we experimented with a range of therapies that chimed better with the times: person-centred therapy, personal construct therapy, rational-emotive therapy, gestalt therapy, and so on. Most of these had the advantage of having been invented by psychologists, and some, at least at their inception, were backed by a healthily respectable body of research. All too soon, of course, these became little more than a mishmash of competing brands, but from them we eventually distilled cognitive behavioural therapy. Even if theoretically self-contradictory, CBT proved to be an ideal combination of behaviourism and cognitivism, and could claim a hopefully impressive scientific pedigree as well as reflecting precisely the popular psychological belief in the individual's freedom to *choose*—in this case to choose a rational belief system from which will follow a serene and ordered life.

There is no doubt that this headlong rush into becoming, essentially, professional therapists did us a lot of good from the purely material aspect of money and status. Clinical psychologists can even become the heroes of TV dramas and documentaries—a sure sign that we have insinuated our way into public awareness in a way that would have been unimaginable forty years ago. It has also brought the mesmerising prospect that, if Lord Layard's fantasies are realised (see for example Layard, 2005) we could become the backbone of a national drive to rid the populace of debilitating and economically unproductive psychological misery. But these achievements have, I think, been bought at a cost—or rather two costs, though they are related.

The first of these is that our scientific role has become paper-thin, almost a figment, existing only as the rigid precepts of what one might call neo-Scientific Management or buried within various so-called 'postmodernist' devices relieving us of the need to take seriously the possibility that there *is* a real world out there. In place of science, we have constructed a kind of theology of method.

The second, related cost is that it has become impossible for many, particularly perhaps younger, clinical psychologists to envisage a role for themselves which would not directly involve making people better. Sooner or later, I fear, it will become all too apparent that there *is* no basis other than self-interest and make-believe for what many of us are supposed to do, just as it will become apparent that it is, indeed, *not* in our power to make people better.

But all is not yet lost. Although CBT threatens to become clinical psychology's defining paradigm, there are still very significant areas of clinical psychological work where its inadequacies are obvious. In situations where people's ability to spin themselves an alternative narrative to disguise their reality is limited, or where the effects of their material circumstances become too obvious to ignore, psychologists (and of course others) are forced to turn their attention to trying to modify the person's world rather than the person's cognitions. This kind of situation is encountered more often in work with people suffering handicaps of body, mind and age (young as well as old) than it is with the kinds of adult mental health problems that tend to have the highest profile in our work. This kind of experience reminds us that there is indeed such a thing as society, and suggests, I think, an alternative to the cognitive-behavioural paradigm, and one which might usefully be extended right across the discipline. All of us exist within a world that is highly resistant to our need, and indeed our desire, to change it. No psychology can hope in the long run to be taken seriously that does not turn outward to the world rather than inward to imagination and discourse. Many clinical psychologists have of course recognised this, but we have yet to discover a paradigm that is sufficiently empirically insistent to give us the confidence to develop a scientific vocabulary to which enough of us can assent; which, in other words, will provide real common ground for us to move forward. But, in principle if not so easily in practice, there is nothing to suggest the task is impossible, and it is perhaps already possible to discern that we shall need to find a vocabulary for talking about social influence on the one hand and embodied subjectivity on the other. In pursuing this task, we wouldn't necessarily have to feel it incumbent on us to 'cure' anyone of anything.

The task itself is of course a conceptual as well as an empirical one. It is also a critical one. Ours is not a green-field site where we can start from scratch with a shiny new edifice, and a great deal may need dismantling before we can even see clearly what lines to take. One of the more irritating objections critics of therapeutic orthodoxy are likely to encounter—as I know only too well—is the demand that critiques have to be coupled with solutions: 'So you say therapy's useless [which, incidentally, I don't], so how would *you* help people.' Critique is groundwork, and particularly difficult—at times even dangerous—because it involves challenging deeply embedded cultural assumptions as well as stubbornly entrenched interests. To insist that critics must have solutions to the problems they try to lay bare is just silly.

One of the greatest difficulties for critics—and indeed seekers after truth in general—is that people's minds are not made up by rational demonstrations of what is the case. This is so as much if not more in academic and professional spheres than it is in everyday life. This is because what people believe is on the whole determined more by Interest than by Reason. How easy it would have been, for example, to clear away the obfuscations caused by the diagnosis 'schizophrenia' if reasoned argument and empirical demonstration were enough to change minds. Challenging received ideas and embedded interests, as for example has Mary Boyle in the case of 'schizophrenia' (Boyle, 2002), takes perseverance, patience, integrity, and maybe even a degree of courage, but in all probability it carries little reward other than serving the cause of truth.

Throughout the history of psychiatry and psychology there have, for example, been those who have been unable to disguise from themselves and others the importance of social factors in the generation of distress. To name just a few of the more obvious ones: Alfred Adler, Erich Fromm, Harry S. Sullivan, Karen Horney, R.D. Laing. But, for all they may enjoy a period of influence and fashionable acceptance, their work invariably ends up as marginal. Few clinical psychology trainees have even heard most of these names, and almost none actually read what they have to say.

What endures is 'magical voluntarism'—or what William Epstein calls 'heroic individualism' (Epstein, 2006). The observation that psychological damage is caused mainly by social structures and relations (pretty obviously true) is always and again hidden behind the idea that individuals choose and control their lives for themselves (pretty clearly false). For every Laing battling the professional establishment there will be a Beck nestling comfortably at its centre. Why? Because it is in our interest that it should be so. If people are not able magically to change their experience of the world, the room in it for therapists becomes a lot less generous.

But the service of truth, philosophically complex though it may be and deeply unfashionable though it is, is no minor cause. Nor, thankfully, is it any longer one that necessarily entails some form of noble self-sacrifice. In fact, in the case of clinical psychology, I think the opposite might well be the case. Unless we rediscover, elaborate and nurture our scientific role—unless, that is, we seek to uncover the truth about what people experience and tell us about their distress—we may well find our profession dribbling away into some constellation of counselling, sociology and politics. Maybe in the greater scheme of things that wouldn't be such a disaster, but it would certainly be a missed opportunity, and, as it happens, the result of a severe miscalculation of where our interests really lie.

REFERENCES

Boyle, M (2002) *Schizophrenia: A scientific delusion?* London: Routledge.
Epstein, W (2006) *Psychotherapy as Religion*. Reno, NV/Las Vegas, NV: University of Nevada Press.
Forshaw, MJ (2007) Free qualitative research from the shackles of method. *The Psychologist, 20,* 478–9.
Jackson, DD (1960) *The Etiology of Schizophrenia*. New York: Basic Books.
Jones, M (1952) *Social Psychiatry*. London: Tavistock.
Layard, R (2005) Therapy for all on the NHS. <http://www.scmh.org.uk/>.
Lidz, T, Fleck, S & Cornelison, A (1965) *Schizophrenia and the Family*. New York: International Universities Press.
Martin, DV (1962) *Adventure in Psychiatry*. Oxford: Cassirer.
Scott, RD & Ashworth, PL (1965) The 'axis value' and the transfer of psychosis. A scored analysis of the interaction in the families of schizophrenic patients. *British Journal of Medical Psychology, 39,* 97–116.

CONTRIBUTORS

PATRICK CALLAGHAN is a Mental Health Nurse and chartered Health Psychologist. He is Professor of Mental Health Nursing at the University of Nottingham, UK, and Nottinghamshire Healthcare NHS Trust where he heads a research programme designed to enable people to recover from mental distress, leading on service evaluation, testing the effects of psychosocial interventions on health and well-being and investigating links between mental health nursing and service user outcomes.

JOCELYN CATTY is a Senior Research Fellow in Mental Health at St. George's, University of London, and a psychodynamic counsellor working in a school and in private practice. Her doctorate was in English Literature and concerned the representation of rape in early modern literature. She has research interests in the interplay between literature and psychoanalysis, as well as in the therapeutic relationship in psychotherapy and psychiatry.

DR. MILES CLAPHAM has trained both as a psychoanalytic psychotherapist with the Philadelphia Association, and as a Child and Adolescent Psychiatrist at Guy's and St Thomas' hospitals in London. He has worked as a Consultant Child and Adolescent Psychiatrist in an NHS Child and Adolescent Mental Health Service for eight years, his native New Zealand for a year, partly in a service for adolescents with early onset psychosis, and a low secure locked adolescent unit for seven years. He moved to St Andrew's Healthcare in Northampton in September 2006, and works 3.5 days a week in the Lowther Adolescent Service, a medium secure psychiatric unit there, currently specialising in young women with a severe level of difficulty, who frequently have a history of early abuse and neglect. He is also based in Cambridge for independent medico-legal work for adolescents, children and their families, and does individual psychotherapy and family based therapeutic work. Dr. Clapham is interested in a philosophical critique of psychotherapy and psychiatry, and in particular is influenced by Wittgenstein's philosophy. He teaches on both the *Introductory Course,* often with colleagues, and on the *Training Course* at the Philadelphia Association. Recent papers were given at the Philosophy, Psychiatry and Psychology Conference in Heidelberg, 2005, the Audit Cultures conference, London, in September 2006, and at the Society for Existential Analysis' Annual Conference, London, on the 'Im/possibilities of Language', in June 2007. He is currently Chair of the Philadelphia Association Trustees, having been on the Training Committee for several years previously.

JOHN CROMBY is a Senior Lecturer in Psychology in the Department of Human Sciences, Loughborough University. He is interested in the way that experience gets produced at the intersection of the body with social influence and studies this intersection by focusing on phenomena such as emotion, 'paranoia', and 'depression'.

BOB DIAMOND works as a clinical psychologist in adult mental health services, Nottingham. He is interested in questioning the limits of existing services in psychiatry and psychotherapy and draws on a critical perspective to establish support that is more meaningful to people experiencing enduring distress.

ALASTAIR MORGAN is a lecturer at the University of Nottingham, UK. He has worked in the mental health field for a number of years, and is also a trained philosopher with a particular interest in Critical Theory and the philosophy of T.W. Adorno. His most recent publication is *Adorno's Concept of Life* (Continuum Press, 2007).

IAN PARKER is Professor of Psychology in the Discourse Unit at Manchester Metropolitan University, where he is managing editor of *Annual Review of Critical Psychology* (<www.discourseunit.com>). His books and articles in the fields of critical psychology, discourse analysis and psychoanalytic theory attempt to connect subjectivity with cultural processes and to possibilities of political change. His most recent book is *Revolution in Psychology: Alienation to Emancipation* (Pluto Press, 2007). Address: Ian Parker, Discourse Unit, Division of Psychology and Social Change, Manchester Metropolitan University, Hathersage Road, Manchester, M13 0JA, UK. Email: <I.A.Parker@mmu.ac.uk>.

DAVID SMAIL was for many years head of Clinical Psychology Services in Nottingham, and held the honorary post of Special Professor in Clinical Psychology at the University of Nottingham until 2000. He retired fully from the NHS in 1998. He is the author of several books on psychotherapy and the social origins of distress, recently *Power, Interest and Psychology* (PCCS Books, 2005). His website is <www.davidsmail.freeuk.com/>.

HELEN SPANDLER is a Research Fellow in the Department of Social Work at the University of Central Lancashire. She is the author of *Asylum to Action: Paddington Day Hospital, Therapeutic communities and beyond* (Jessica Kingsley Publishers, 2006), and co-editor (with Sam Warner) of *Beyond Fear and Control: Working with young people who self harm* (A 42nd Street reader) (PCCS Books, 2007).

PHILIP THOMAS is Professor of Philosophy, Diversity and Mental Health in the Institute for Philosophy, Diversity and Mental Health at the Centre for Ethnicity and Health in the University of Central Lancashire. He is also chair of *Sharing Voices Bradford*, a community development project working with Bradford's Black and Minority Ethnic communities. After working as a full-time consultant psychiatrist in the NHS for over twenty years, he left clinical practice in 2004 to focus on writing and academic work. His academic interests include philosophy (post-structuralism and critical theory), and their application to psychiatry, especially social and cultural psychiatry, psychology and medicine. He is also interested in narrative and the moral and ethical problems of representation in medicine and literature. He is particularly interested in the practical value of narrative in 'recovery' from psychosis. He has developed alliances with survivors of psychiatry, service users and community groups, locally, nationally and internationally, and is well known for the column he wrote with his colleague Pat Bracken in *Open Mind* magazine, called *Postpsychiatry*. He is a founder member and co-chair of the Critical Psychiatry Network in Britain. He has published well over 100 scholarly papers. Free Association Books published his first book, *Dialectics of Schizophrenia*, in 1997. His second book *Voices of Reason, Voices of Insanity* written with Ivan Leudar and published by Brunner-Routledge in April 2000, examined the different meanings attached to the experience of hearing voices over 2,500 years of Western culture. Oxford University Press published his third book, *Postpsychiatry*, co-authored with Pat Bracken, in 2005.

CHRISTOPHER D. WARD is Professor and Consultant in Neurological Medicine, working primarily with long-term and progressive neurological disorders. He also has a specialist role in a service for people with chronic fatigue syndrome. He is currently exploring the relevance of systemic family therapy in these fields.

DAVE R. WILSON is a Mental Health Lecturer at the University of Nottingham. He is the programme lead for the 'BS (Hons) in Mental Health and Social Care (Forensic)'. His previous clinical experience includes a decade as a Forensic Community Psychiatric Nurse, three years as a Charge Nurse on what used to be called a 'Challenging Behaviour' ward, as well as having worked on Acute Psychiatric Admission wards. He also spent a number of years working as a Nursing Assistant working with the elderly mentally ill. Other reasonably long-term jobs have included work as an art teacher, a painter and decorator, a postman, and he also spent most of his not-so-callow youth in the Royal Marines.

He is a trained sculptor, a published poet (one piece in one anthology), and has a degree in Aesthetic Education. His interests include the Visual Arts (all of them), Philosophy (Existentialism and Phenomenology), and he has a profound weakness for Sci-Fi and Western movies. His current research interests are around non-verbal communication, perception, and something called 'thin-slicing'.
He says that his greatest achievements are being married for nearly thirty years and being a father to two for over twenty years.

SUSANNAH WILSON has a Modern languages background, and did a first degree and MA at Manchester University in French Studies. She completed a DPhil in Modern Languages at the University of Oxford in 2005 on the subject of writing by psychiatric patients in France in the period 1850–1920. Her research interests lie in the areas of gender, autobiography and the history of psychiatry in France. Her thesis is in the process of being published with Oxford University Press under the working title of *Voices from the Asylum: Four French women writers, 1850–1920*.

INDEX

A

Acocella, J 141, 148
Adler, A 196
Adorno, TW 10, 11, 55, 60, 64, 65, 69
aesthetics 72, 160
Afuape, T 179, 187
Alaszewski, A 91, 96
Aletheia 76
alienation 160, 176
'alienist' 99, 100, 104
Allbutt, TA 132, 134, 135, 136
Alloy, LB 141, 148
American Psychiatric Association (APA) 37, 148
anarchy 92, 93
Andreasen, N 26, 27, 28, 29, 30, 37
André-Thomas, 136
animals 4, 45–6
Anthony, WA 55, 69
anthropomorphising, cultural practice of 45
antidepressants 78
anti-psychiatric
   alternatives, critique of 91
   initiatives 84
anti-psychiatrists 87
   feminists have criticised 91
anti-psychiatry 92
   figures 88
anti-racist, feminist work 42
Antoine, G 101, 109
Ardrey, R 156, 171, 172
Arnold, M 130, 131, 132, 136
Aronson, R 160, 172
Artaud, A 9, 138–9, 144, 147, 148
   life and work 138
Asch, S 153
Asen, E 125, 136
Ashworth, PL 190, 196
asylum/s 26, 99, 100, 101, 105, 106, 108
Athanasou, JA 146, 149
Attention Deficit Hyperactivity Disorder (ADHD) 175

Attides, Louis des 139
Augustine, St. 35, 118, 123
autism 26, 28

B

Bacon, Francis 164
Baerveldt, C 17, 22
Bain, A 126, 127, 128, 129, 130, 132, 136
Baldwin, C 30, 36, 37
Ballet, G 125, 127, 128, 133, 136
Barker, P 55, 69
Barkstead, W 115, 123
Baron, C 84, 91, 92, 93, 96
Barrett, R 25, 37
Barthes, R 42, 51, 52
Bartky, SL 112, 123
Bataille, G 63, 69
Baudelaire, C 64, 139, 147
Baudrillard, J 159, 165, 170, 172
Beckett, Samuel 139
behaviour
   erratic 141
   harmful 141
   therapy unscientific 194
   unorthodox 142
   verbal 27, 153, 155
being-in-the-world 5, 13, 32, 62, 159
'being-with' 162
beliefs 17
Benjamin, W 63, 64, 69
Benner, P 156, 172
Bennett, MR 73, 82
Bentall, R 54, 69, 140, 144, 148, 177, 188
Berger, J 79, 80, 82, 168, 172
Bergson, H 60, 61, 63, 69
Berrios, G 135, 136
Bible, the Good News 131, 136
Bilevsky, D 49, 52
Binswanger, L 55
biochemistry 127–8
bio-electricity 127
biomedical model 143, 174, 190

INDEX

Blackman, L 14, 22, 25, 37, 43, 52
Bleuler, E 26, 37
Block, J 22, 23
bodily
   economy, the 128
   senses, feedback from 13
   shame 112
body
   dysmorphic disorder (BDD) 112
   mind and 116, 123, 143, 160
Bonar, H 131
Booth, R 50, 52
Bostock, J 181, 182, 183, 185, 187
boundary/ies 44
   between
      health and illness 44
      human beings and animals 45
      masculinity and femininity 46, 86
      normality and pathology 8, 50, 51
      reason and madness 42
   changes 45–6, 50
   crossing 90, 91
Bourdieu, P 15, 22
Bouricius, J 25, 36, 37
Bouté, G 107, 109
Boyle, M 178, 187, 195, 196
Bracken, P 11, 25, 32, 37
Brison, S 25, 37
British Broadcasting Corporation (BBC) 148
British Psychological Society (BPS) 145
Brown, G 113, 114, 123
Brown, T 87, 96
Bruner, J 21, 22
Buddhist doctrine of 'no mind' 74
Burman, E 46, 52
Burnard, P 152, 172
Burston, D 85, 96
Burstow, B 91, 96
Burton, AK 144, 145, 150
Burton, M 178, 180, 187
business
   ideology 191
   mind 192
   view 192
Butler, J 57, 69

C

Callaghan, P 9, 145, 148
Campbell, P 86, 93, 96
Capgras, J 101, 102, 109
capitalist society 2, 41, 65, 66
Carper, B 165, 172
Carr, D 31, 37
Cartesian
   dualism 160
   split between subject and object 20
Cassar, J 106, 109
Castel, R 99, 109
Catty, J 8, 114, 119, 123
Chalmers, DJ 162, 172
Charenton, asylum at 101, 102, 104
charismatic leader 84, 85, 91, 94
Charlton, B 175, 187
Chatterton Dix, W 131
children 76, 175
Chipp, HB 163, 172
chronic fatigue syndrome (CFS) 9, 125, 126, 128, 133, 134, 136
   realness of 135
Churchyard, T 116, 123
Clare, A 140, 148
Clare, John 147
Claudel, C 100, 101, 106–7
Claudel, Paul 106
coercion 3
cognitive
   behaviour therapy (CBT) 71, 78, 81, 82, 184, 194, 195
   psychology 17
cognitivist models, dominance of 9
Cohen, D 21, 23
Cohen de Lara-Kroon, N 43
Coleman, R 25, 37, 184, 187
Coles, R 95, 96
communication 27, 64, 152
   hysteria as 134
   phatic 152, 158
communities 182
community
   psychology 181, 182, 183
   therapeutic, movement in psychiatry 85, 88, 91, 93 ,190
complementary medicine 191
compulsion 2, 3
consciousness 6, 61, 63, 64, 67, 75, 81, 111, 162, 178
   -raising 43
context, particularity of 8, 41–2
Cooper, D 87, 88, 94, 96
Corin, E 34, 37
counter-transference 80, 81

Court Assessment Team 152
Crellin, C 45, 52
Cresswell, M 86, 96
Creuzet, P 128, 133, 136
Crighton, DA 166, 173
critical
    perspective 24
    psychology 181, 186,
    realist framework 177–9
    Theory 64, 174
    thinking 174
Cromby, J 7, 15, 16, 19, 21, 22, 177, 187
Crossley, M 25, 38
Crossley, N 38, 86, 87, 96
Crow, T 27, 38
Cummins, JJ 131

D

Damasio, AR 14, 17, 22
Daniel, S 115, 123
Davidson, L 25, 28, 30, 38
Davis, K 178, 189
de la Chapelle, A 107, 109
Deegan, P 55, 69
Delbée, A 106, 109
Deleuze, G 63, 69
demonic despair 77
Department of Health (DH) 55, 69, 144, 146, 148
    and Social Security 172
Depraz, N 163, 172
depression 77, 78, 79, 125, 146, 147
derailment (positive thought disorder) 27
Derrida, J 13, 22
Descartes, R 159, 160
    Window 159
Deschamps, A 129, 136
despair 77, 141, 177, 178, 187
    demonic 77
    more than depression 77
Diagnostic & Statistical Manual (DSM) 140, 142, 190
    criticisms of the 143
diagnostic labelling 54, 142
Diamond, R 9, 176, 180, 182, 183, 187
Dickinson, E 147
Dilthey, W 28, 60, 61, 69
Dineen, T 176, 177, 184, 187
discourse analysis 42
display rules 15

divorce 100
doctor–patient relationship 79, 80
Donaldson, I 119, 123
Dostoevsky, FM 140, 149
Doty, WG 85, 86, 91, 92, 93, 96, 97
Double, D 174, 187
Douieb, B 90
Downs, J 183, 187
Drayton, M 116, 123
drug treatments, promoting 175
Dubois, P 136
durée, concept of 63
Durkin, L 89, 96

E

ecstasy 21
Edge, I 183, 187
Edmeston, J 131
Ehrenreich, B 145, 149
Einstein, A 73, 74
    metaphor
        to describe the study of the mind 73
        for the object of physics 73
Ekman, P 15, 22
emotion/s 13, 14
    expression of 15
    social construction of 45
    theories 15
emotional
    extra- feelings 14, 15
    inappropriate reactions 141
employment 144, 145, 183
energy in Victorian biology 126
Epstein, WM 175, 184, 187, 196
Erfahrung 59, 60, 64
Erlebnis 59, 60, 61, 63, 64
Escher, S 184, 188
Esslin, M 138, 148, 149
ethical
    mental health work 55
    narrativity 31
    problem in mental health care 3
    ways of thinking about narrative in psychology 25
ethics 72, 77, 78
    code of 79
    importance of 77
    of psychiatry 68
Eugenics movement 190
European Union (EU) 146, 149

Evans, EP 45, 52
evidence
    -based medicine 78
    based on facts 6
    and practice 174
    supporting the services 175
experience/s 59, 60, 67
    concept of 59
    epistemic and normative claims of lived 56
    of everyday life 66
    expertise from 66
    failure of words to articulate 33
    limits of, Hegel overturns Kantian 60
    of madness 67
    ownership of 66
    qualitative approach to understanding 54
    of service users 58
    transcendent 66
    what it means to have an 57
extra-
    conscious
        elements 6
        experience 5
    -emotional feelings 14, 15
eye/s
    becomes a window on the world outside 159
    contact 151, 168
    as interior-exterior arbitrator 161
    Judas, The 154, 155, 159, 164, 165, 166, 167
    perceiving, the 161
    Phenomenologist's, The 160
    -to-eye encounter 162
Eysenck, Hans 193
Ezriel, H 89
Ezzy, D 146, 149

F

Faber, FW 131
family romance scenario 101
Fanon, F 179, 187
fantasy 34
fatigue 128, 130
    the mental physiology of 128
    as metaphor 133
    moral 130
        dimension of medical 132
    in tissues and organs 126
    or weariness 125

Faulkner, William 147
Fauvel, A 100, 109
Featherstone, B 93, 98
feedback from our bodily senses 13
feeling traps 19
    are inherently relational 20
feelings 12
    emotional 13
    of knowing 14, 15
felt body 13
female
    complaint 111
        and sexual shame 113
    psychiatrists 94
    tricksters figures 86
femininity 46
    historical association with madness 45
feminist/s 91
    anti-psychiatrists, criticism of 91
    anti-racist work 42
    movement 43
Fernie, E 113, 119, 123
first impressions 154
First Person Narratives (FPNs) 25
Fiumara, GC 80, 82
Fleck, S 196
Flykt, A 21, 23
Forshaw, MJ 192, 196
Foucault, M 3, 9, 11, 25, 26, 33, 38, 42, 43, 44, 50, 52, 57, 63, 68, 69, 139, 140, 141, 144, 149, 179, 187
Frankfurt School 63, 65
Fraser, WI 26, 39
Freedman, B 155, 162, 167, 172
freedom 65, 66, 87
    concept of 63
Freeman, J 87, 91, 96
Freud, S 54, 64, 71, 73, 74, 75, 80, 101, 109, 112, 123, 127, 135, 136, 151, 164
    description of shame 112
Fromm, E 196
Fryer, D 145, 183, 187
Fryers, T 21, 23
Fulford, B 163, 172

G

Gadamer, H-G 60, 69
Galen 144
Gardner, H 178, 189
Gaudichon, B 106, 108, 109

gaze 162, 167, 168, 170
   into an abyss 170
   non-threatening 168
   Valery's model of 162
General Health Questionnaire (GHQ) 146
Genet, Jean 139
Georgaca, E 50, 52, 97, 149
gestalt psychotherapy 85
Gilbert, P 112, 123
Gladwell, M 154, 155, 164, 172
glance 153
Glass, JM 17, 22
Glendinning, S 162, 172
globalisation 41
Goffman, E 86, 96
Goldstein, J 99, 109

Goodburn, J 8, 88, 89, 90, 91, 92, 93, 94
   as Trickster 88
Goodman, CC 21, 22
Gordo López, AJ 40, 52
government 175
Goya 144
grammar of life 75
Gray, D 28, 38
Greene, M 140, 149
Greenhalgh, T 24, 38
Guattari, F 69
Guevara, Che 148
guilt and shame, distinction between 111
Gunnell, D 21, 22

H

Habermas 67
Hacker, PMS 73, 82
Haddon, B 91, 96
Hagan, T 186, 188
hallucinations 20
Hanvey, C 87, 96
happiness 3
Harper, D 19, 21, 22, 52, 184, 188
Harré, R 45, 52
Harrison, G 21, 22
Hartman, D 85, 98
Healthcare Commission 79
hearing voices 27
   Network 183
Heath, I 24, 38
Heaton, J 71, 72, 73, 75, 79, 81, 82
Hegel, GWF 59, 60, 69

   overturns the Kantian limits of
      experience 60
   philosophy 55, 59
Heidegger, M 5, 31, 38, 61, 62, 63, 69, 76, 81, 83, 168, 172
Helen of Troy 115
Henle, M 153, 172
Herder, JG 61
hermeneutic approach 10
heroic individualism 196
Hillman, J 140, 149
Hinshelwood, RD 91, 96
history, particularity of 43
Hobson, RF 85, 96
Holland, S 180, 183, 188
Holmes, J 24, 38
Hook, D 51, 52
Hopkins, Gerard Manley 147
Horney, K 196
Hornstein, G 25, 38
Hotopf, M 133, 137
housing 183
Hovell, D de Berdt 126, 136
Howell, T 113, 123
human
   being 7
      is fundamentally historical 31
      existence, particularity of 6
      and a feeling body 12
      potentialities defined in terms of functioning 3
HUMAN project 12
   concern with mental health 17
   research group 1
   research project 1
humour 85, 89, 91
Hurwitz, B 24, 38
Husserl, E 61, 63, 69, 168
Hyde, L 85, 86, 88, 89, 90, 91, 94, 97
Hydén, L-C 28, 38
Hymns Ancient & Modern Revised 131, 136
Hynes, WJ 85, 86, 89, 91, 92, 93, 96, 97

I

ideas, mistaken 72
identity, connection between shame and 113
idols 164, 166
   enslave our thought 164
imagery 34
Immelman, A 52

individual 184
  psychological help 184
  responsibility 184
Ingleby, D 67, 69
International Classification of Diseases (ICD-10) 140, 143
  and *DSM*, criticisms of the 143
interpretation 171
interview room/s 152, 158
Irvine, AH 162, 172
isolation 18, 160, 176

J

Jackson, DD 190, 196
Jahoda, M 145
James, W 14, 22
Jameson, F 164
Jansen, A 21, 22
Jaspers, K 2, 4, 5, 6, 11, 25, 38, 54
Jay, M 60, 63, 69, 164, 171, 172
Jenner, FA 84, 97
Jimenez-Dominguez, BH 178, 188
Johnson, RE 165, 172
Johnstone, E 26, 38
Johnstone, L 12, 18, 19, 20, 22, 176, 188
Jones, E 125, 136
Jones, M 190, 196
Jong, E 92, 97
Jove (Roman god) 118
Jung, CG 85, 86, 97, 109

K

Kagan, C 180, 183, 188
Kant, I 59, 60, 70
  philosophy 59, 62
Keats, John 132, 136
Kempe, Margery 25
Kennard, D 85, 97
Kierkegaard, S 76, 77, 83
Kihlstrom, JF 154, 155, 164, 165, 172
Killen, A 134, 136
King Lear 141, 148
Klerman, G 26, 38
Knight, T 184, 188
knowing of the 'third kind' 14
Kopp, S 85, 97
Kraepelin, E 26
Kurtz, S 173

L

Lacan, J 76, 81, 83
Laing, RD 28, 38, 79, 85, 88, 91, 94, 190, 196
Lam, JA 145, 149
Langer, S 13, 14, 23
language 26, 72, 75, 76, 78, 80, 81
  act of reclaiming 25
  human use of 75
  interrogation of 71
  limits of logic and 72
  ordinary chat 152
  primacy of 34
  of psychiatry 26
  psychotherapeutic 81
  scientific 72
  theory of 74
  therapeutic 80
    possibilities and limits of 80
  and truth, relationship between 76
Lauer, G 169
Launer, J 24, 38
Lauzon, G 34, 37
Layard, R 184, 188, 194, 196
Le Normant des Varannes, E 101
Leda (Roman godess) 118
Leder, D 16, 23
Leitner, M 85, 97
Lenin, Vladimir 51
Lethe (river of forgetfulness) 76
Levin, DM 159, 164, 173
Levy, R 112, 123
Lewis, Sir A 140
Lewis, HB 19, 23, 111, 123
Lewis, M 111, 1117, 123, 141
Lidz, T 190, 196
life
  everyday critique of 65
  experience of everyday 66
  grammar of 75
  philosophy, or *Lebensphilosophie* 60, 61
Lin, TY 149
lived experience 54, 55, 56
  authority of 68
  concept of 59
  epistemic and normative claims of 56
  philosophical history of concept of 56
  positivism of 56
  three forms of 66
Lloyd, A 137

logic and language, limits of 72
Lomas, P 184, 188
Lorde, A 91, 97
Lordi (Finnish pop group) 48, 49, 50
Lucrece 110, 115, 116, 117, 118, 119, 120
    shame and suicide 118
    story 118
Lukács, G 65, 70
Lynch, T 175, 188

M

MacIntyre, A 31, 38
madness 140, 141, 142
    and the absence of work 144–8
    classifying 142
    and destruction of creativity 146
    experience of 67
    in the 15th century 25
    four forms of 141
    historically associated with femininity 45
    history of 44
    the nature of 139
    perspectives on 142
    postmodern perspective of 142
    by romantic identification 141
    and the self, relationship between 67
    silencing of 26
magic and make-believe 191
magical voluntarism 196
magistrate/'s 152
    cells 153
    staff 152
Maitland, S 34, 38
Makarius, L 87, 93, 97
Malinowski, B 152, 173
Manthorpe, J 91, 96
Marcuse, H 64
Martin, DV 190, 196
Martin-Baro, Ignacio 178
Mason, M 126, 137
Masson, J 184, 188
Matheson, G 131
Matilda 115
May, R 184, 188
McCole, J 64, 70
McHugh, P 2, 11
McLaughlin, T 50, 52, 97, 149
McLean, C 164, 149
meaning exists in the absence of words 24

medical
    and biological paradigms 175
    director, role of 89
    model of illness 125
    perspective 142
medicalisation of children's behaviour 175
medication, psychotropic, effects of 174
medicine 24, 78
    treats physical illness as a model 4
Meltzer, H 185, 188
Melucci, A 87, 97
Melzer, D 21, 23
mental
    disorder across cultures 141
    distress
        a product of being human 4
        severe 5, 7, 158
    health
        assessment 169
        concept of 40
        as cultural practice 40
        methodology used to study 40
        Officer (MHO) 151, 152, 158, 161, 165, 168
        services, using 180, 183
    illness, myth of 86
    patients' unions 90, 93
mentalism 75
Merleau-Ponty, M 13, 17, 20, 23, 61, 62, 70, 167
Merriman, JM 102, 109
metaplay 89
methodological
    individualism 9
    requirements 40
Meyer, C 14, 23
Mezan, P 85, 97
Michaelson, J 176, 189
Miller, DL 160, 173
Miller, P 91, 97
Mills, C Wright 136, 137
mind, the 72, 73, 74
    and body 160
    known only to the individual 72
    picture of the 72
    scientific understanding of the 72
Minkowski, E 55
Mirowsky, J 21, 23
models of recovery 55
Mollon, P 112, 114, 122, 123
Moloney, P 175, 188

Moncrieff, J 21, 23, 174, 188
Moneiro, ACD 97
Moomins, The 41
Moominvalley 41
moral
   dimension of medical fatigue 132
   fatigue 130
   practical- knowledge 14
Moran, D 162, 167, 168, 173
Moreau de Tours, J-J 100, 109
Morgan, A 65, 70
Morrison, Jim 139
Morrissey, J 145, 148
Mosher, LR 85, 97
Mosso, A 129, 137
Mullan, B 91, 97
Munch, Edvard 147
Murat, L 100, 109
Murphy, GC 146, 149
music 34, 37, 41, 139
mute 28
myth of mental illness 86

N

Nagel, T 151, 173
Napoleonic Civil Code 100
narrative/s 24, 26, 55, 195
   absence of 25
   approach to illness 24
   challenge our conception of 37
   critique of the 31
   danger of 30
   expression, forms of 37
   importance in psychiatry 24
   and important ethical purpose 24
   loss 25, 30
      temporary 30
         schizophrenia and 28
   of madness 25
   narrator and, relationship between 32
   non- people 31
   of people's lives 24
   in psychology, ethical ways of thinking
      about 25
   in psychosis 25
   schizophrenia, psychopathology and 26
   of self-experience 57
   and selfhood 31
narrativity
   thesis, criticism of the ethical 33
   ethical 31
   psychological 31
National Institute for Health and Clinical
   Excellence (NICE) 78, 79, 175, 177
Neale, JM 131
Nelson, G 178, 181, 188
neo-Kraepelinism 26, 27
neurasthenia 9, 125, 126, 127, 128, 133
   biological basis of 126
   and Chronic Fatigue Syndrome 133, 134
neurogenetics 73
neuromechanics 127
neuroscience 129
   modern 73
Newton, J 144, 149
Nichterlein, Maria 51
Nietzsche, F 60, 61, 170, 173
Nightingale, D 177, 187
Nissinen, T 48
'no mind', Zen Buddhist concept of 74
non-judgemental 9
   attitude 9
Norton, K 90, 97
noun 74
   abstract 74
   concrete 74
   distinction between concrete and abstract
      74
   'schizophrenia' is laden with meanings
      25
Novalis, 61
Nuytten, B 106, 109

O

O'Neill, Eugene 147
Ohman, A 21, 23
Oppenheim, J 134, 137
oppression, axes of 44
Orcs (in *The Lord of the Rings*) 48
Owen, K 146, 149

P

Paddington Day Hospital 8, 84, 88, 90, 92
Painter, W 119, 123
Palmer, RE 61, 70
panic button 152
Paris, R-M 109
Parker, I 7, 40, 43, 46, 50, 51, 52, 91, 92,
   97, 112, 140, 143, 149

Parker, R 112, 123
Parkin, G 187
Pascal, Blaise 140
patient/s 79
    doctor and, relationship between 79
    female, writing by 100
Patterson, P 153, 173
Paulhan, Jean 147
Pembroke, L 37, 38
Perkins, R 55, 70, 144, 149
persons, theory of 72
pharmaceutical industry 175, 190
phenomenological
    attitude 163, 167
    critique of psychology and psychiatry 76
phenomenology 54, 55, 61, 62, 63, 64, 162, 163
    issues of perception and meaning 159–62
Philadelphia Association (PA) 79
Phillips, J 29, 31, 32, 34, 38
philosophical
    history of the concept of lived experience 56
    theories about the nature of selfhood 31
philosophy 28, 71
    intersection of psychopathology and 28
    of life or *Lebensphilosophie* 60
    as a therapy 72
Phoenix, A 42, 52
Pilgrim, D 93, 97, 142, 149, 176, 177, 180, 188
Pinel, P 99
Pines, M 112, 113, 123
Plath, Sylvia 147
Poe, Edgar Allan 139
poetic and religious visions of weariness 130
poetry 34, 37, 147
    Elizabethan 8
    Victorian 130
postmodern pragmatism 7
Potter, J 42, 52
poverty 183
    of speech 28, 30, 35
        content 28
power 42, 156, 174, 176, 182, 183
    mapping 186
    relationships 91
    professional, devolve 183
powerlessness 156
pragmatics 27
prejudice 162, 166, 167

pre-verbal relational dyad/s 168, 171
Pribesh, S 21, 23
Prilleltensky, I 178, 180, 181, 188
privilege, positions of 179
psychiatric
    drug treatments, promoting 175
    practice 84
        resistance to 86
psychiatrist 90
    anti-, term 87, 88
        critique of 91
    female 94
    paradox of 87
    radical 85, 92
    as trickster, limitations of the 90
psychiatry 2, 54, 68
    abuses of 68
    anti- 88, 91, 92
    central concepts for 6
    critiques of 8
    democratic 95
    disappearance of 3
    ethics of 68
    horizons for understanding 4
    language of 26
    and a medical paradigm 2
    major elements of 54
    profession of 175
    role of 26
    scientific 26
    therapeutic community movement in 190
psychoanalysis 54
psychodynamic theorist 72
psychological
    accounts of shame, and psychoanalytic 110
    help 184
    narrativity 31
    perspectives 142
    practice, transparent 177, 182
psychologism 75
    criticising 73
psychologists
    as pawns 176
    vested interests and 177
psychology
    community, salient principles of 182
    dominance of Western 179
    plant 45
    a questioning 180–2, 184, 186

psychopathology 4, 26, 28
    and philosophy, intersection of 28
    relationship between unemployment and 146
    schizophrenia and narrative 26
psychosis
    debates about 25
    severe 24
psychotherapeutic language 81
psychotherapy
    as civil religion 175
    efficacy of 184
    gestalt 85
psychotic 'hieroglyphic' speech and actions 28
psychotropic medication, effects of 174
Putin, Vladimir 49

Q

questioning psychology, a 180–2, 184, 186

R

Radin, P 85, 86, 94, 97
rape
    association between shame and 110
    and seduction, difference between 114
rating scales, Andreasen's 29
reality contact 141
reason 42, 50, 58, 60, 144, 192
reconstructing the self following trauma 25
recovery 24, 25
    models of 55
    from psychosis 25
    from schizophrenia 28
        debarred from 25
Reed, Jeremy 147, 149
Reed, Jim 176, 188
Reeves, WC 133, 137
reflective, capacity to be 30
rehabilitation 24
reification, concept of 65
relationship between
    doctor and patient 79
    language and truth 76
    madness and the self 67
    narrator and narrative 32
    unemployment and psychopathology 146
religion/s
    fundamentalist 191

psychotherapy being a civil 175
religious visions of weariness and oblivion 130–2
Repper, J 55, 70, 144, 149
repression 75
research 183, 190
    feminist 44
    problematic issues in qualitative 42
    psychiatric 6
    qualitative 40, 43, 44, 51
Reynolds, J 176, 188
Riadore, JE 134, 137
Richardson, BW 130, 132, 137
Rickman, HP 70
Ricoeur, P 31, 38
Rigoli, J 100, 109
Rilke, Rainer Maria 147
Rimbaud, Arthur 147
risk, assessment of to self 151, 169
Ritalin 175
Ritsher, JEB 21, 23
Rivière, A 106, 108, 109, 139, 147
Roberts, G 24, 38
Robertson, R 41, 53
Rodez Asylum 139
Rodin, Auguste 106, 107
Roe, D 25, 28, 30, 38
Roethke, T 170, 173
Rogers, A 93, 97, 142, 149, 176, 188
Romme, M 184, 188
Rorschach blot images 43
Rosaldo, MS 112, 123
Rosamond 115, 116
Rose, G 84, 97
Rose, N 91, 97, 179, 188
Rosenheck, R 145, 149
Ross, CE 21, 23
Rossetti, C 131, 132, 137
Rothenburg, A 147, 149
Routledge, P 88, 97
Rouy, Hersilie 100, 101, 107, 108, 109
Ruthrof, H 16, 23
Ryle, G 73, 83

S

Sachs, J 146, 149
Sacks, H 158
sadomasochism 15
Sainsbury Centre for Mental Health [SCMH] 144, 149

210

Salpêtrière, the women's public asylum 101
Sampson, EE 13, 23
samurai 46
  sword 47
  in images of madness 46
Sartre, JP 160, 161, 162, 171, 173
sauvages 141
Savage, G 135, 137
Savill, TD 125, 127, 130, 137
Sawacki, J 44, 53
Scarry, E 16, 23
Scheff, T 19, 23
Scheler, M 166, 173
Schelling, FWJ 61
Schiller, F 61
schizophrenia 24, 25, 67
  clinical features of 25
  debarred from recovery 25
  key symptom of 26
  and narrative loss 28
  noun is laden with meanings 25
  psychopathology and narrative 26
  and silence, challenges to 34
  symptoms of 27
Schlosser, E 146, 149
Schnädelbach, H 61, 70
Schneider, Kurt 54, 55
science 72
  contribution to understanding 72
scientific
  enquiry 192, 193
  language 72
  psychiatry 26
  understanding of the mind 72
Scott, JW 56, 70
Scott, RD 190, 196
Seedhouse, D 158, 164, 173
Seider, S 178, 189
self, the 73
  -harm 77
  -understandings 6
selfhood
  and narrative 31–4
  in psychosis 25, 26, 28, 30, 31
Sellin, E 139, 149
Semelaigne, R 99, 109
Sérieux, P 101, 102, 109
serotonin-specific reuptake inhibitors (SSRIs) 21
Serrano-Garcia, I 183, 189

service user/s
  experiences of 54, 58, 67
  movement 93
  narratives of 56
  views 58
sexual
  abuse 112, 114
    the ultimate shame 112
  politics 91
  shame 110, 111, 113–14, 116, 122
sexuality 75, 76
Shakespeare, William 110, 117, 119, 124
  Lucrece 110, 111, 118–20
shame (see also sexual shame) 8
  association between rape and 110
  bodily 112
  connection between identity and 113
  defined 111
  in Elizabethan poetry 121
  and guilt, distinction between 111
  and identity 111
  mirrors of 115
  private 113
  -proneness as a pathology 110
  psychological and psychoanalytic accounts of 110
  public 113
  root of the word 111
  and shaming today 120
  spectacle of 117
shaming, acts of 8, 112
Sharpe, M 133, 137
Shedler, J 22, 23
Shepherd, C 133, 137
Shingler, A 37, 38
Shores wife 115
Shorter, E 134, 135, 137
Shortt, SED 146, 149
Shotter, J 13, 14, 23
Showalter, E 91, 92, 97, 134, 137
Sidlauskas, S 159, 173
silence 25, 30, 34
  approach to 34
  and meaning 34
silencing of madness 26
Silverman, J 154, 173
Simon, B 140, 149
Simpson, J 16, 23
Sinclair, J 126, 137
Smail, D 9, 22, 23, 175, 179, 184, 185, 186, 188, 189

Smeets, T 21, 22
Smith, H 50, 52
social
   construction of emotion 45
   injustices 183
   and material contexts, link 185
Sokolowski, R 159, 162, 173
Solzhenitsyn, Alexander 164
Sontag, Susan 133, 137
Spandler, H 8, 84, 87, 88, 89, 90, 91, 92, 93, 97
speech, poverty of 28, 30, 35
Spencer, H 126, 127, 128, 130, 137
spermatorrhoea 126
Stalin, Joseph 51
Stanley, L 43, 53
Sterling, D 145, 149
Stevens, Wallace 164
Stewart, A 183, 187
stigma 3, 158
Stone, B 33, 39
Stowell Smith, M 50, 52, 97
Strachey, J 151
Strawson, G 31, 32, 33, 39
Strindberg, August 147
Stroll, A 72, 83
suffering caused by mistaken ideas 72
suicide 146
Sullivan, HS 196
supernatural perspective 142
survivor movement 25
Swain, G 99, 109
Swinburne, AC 131, 132, 137
symptoms 135
   meanings of 135
   negative 27
   positive 27
   Schedule for the Assessment of Negative 29
Szasz, T 86, 94

T

Tangney, JP 112, 124
Tannen, RS 86, 94, 98
Taylor, C 35, 39
technology 6, 190
Tennyson, Alfred Lord 132, 137
tests, projective 43
Thatcher, Margaret 190, 191
   /Reagan counter-revolution 190

therapeutic
   community movement in psychiatry 190
   conversations, supportive and 185
   encounters 8
   language 80
Theseus 118
thin-slicing 154, 167
Thiselton, AC 169, 173
Thomas, P 6, 11, 25, 26, 27, 32, 37, 39
Thomas, T 89, 98
Thomson, JA 130, 137
thought
   disorder (TD) 25, 26
      negative 27
      positive 27
   Language and Communication Scale (TLC) 27
Timimi, S 175, 189
Towl, GJ 166, 173
transcendent experiences 66
transcendental epoché 61, 63
transference 81
transparency 178
Tranströmer, Tomas 24, 39
Trappists 36
Trélat, U 101, 109
trickster
   figures 8, 86, 87
      female 86, 94
      from world mythology 85, 88
   Goodburn as 88–90
   healer 85
   limitations of the psychiatrist as 90–2
   positive force 84
   stories of radical failure 92–4
Trussell, J 117, 124
Tseng, WS 141, 149

U

unconscious 76, 164
   adaptive 164, 165
   at work 154
   no place for the 76
unemployment and psychopathology, relationship between 146
United Nations (UN) 146, 149
Ussher, J 46, 53

V

Valéry, P 162, 167
　model of the gaze 162
Van Gogh, Vincent 144, 147
Vernon, MD 165, 173
Victorian poetry 130
Voestermans, P 17, 22
voices, people who hear 27, 183
Vonnegut, Kurt 178, 189
Vygotsky, LS 16, 23

W

Waddell, G 144, 145, 150
Wakefield, JC 141
Waldron, L 180, 188
Wall, W 113, 124
Wallcraft, J 176, 189
Waller, G 14, 23
Walsh, M 91, 96
Warner, R 86, 98
Warner, V 21, 23
Warr, P 146, 150
Wartegg, E 43
Waters, A 14, 23
Watson, N 146, 149
Watts, A 74, 83
Weille, KL 15, 23
Weiner, DB 109
Welch, S 146, 150
Wells, L 29, 39
Wessely, S 133, 137
White, S 84, 88, 90, 91, 93, 94, 95, 98, 165, 173
Whittington, R 153, 173
Wiedenbach, E 156, 173
Williams, R 14, 15, 23
Williams, Tennessee 147
Wilson, C 160, 173
Wise, S 43, 53
Wittgenstein, L 8, 71, 72, 73, 74, 76, 78, 80, 82, 83
　notion of language games 73
　philosophy 72
Wolpe, Joseph 193
women/'s
　health 183
　incarcerated in asylums 8
　tricksters 86, 94
Woody, M 33, 34, 37, 39

Woolston, C 146, 147, 150
words 24
　failure of to articulate experience 33
　meaning exists in the absence of 24
work 144
　absence of 138, 144, 146
　　and madness 144, 146
　confers status and identity 145
　promotes recovery 145
　provides a means of structuring and occupying 145
Worker's Hall of Tampere 51
working class 44
World Health Organisation (WHO) 134, 143, 150
world music 41
Wright Mills, C 178, 189
Wroe, S 49, 53
Wurmser, L 111, 112, 124

Y

Yuval-Davis, N 44, 53

Z

Zeldin, T 100, 109
Zimberoff, D 85, 98
Zukav, G 73, 83

Lightning Source UK Ltd.
Milton Keynes UK
UKHW021855161220
375374UK00003B/144